Overcoming Common Problems

Coping with Perimenopause

Janet Wright

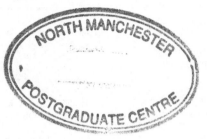

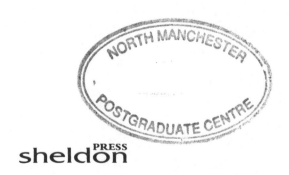

sheldon **PRESS**

First published in Great Britain in 2006

Sheldon Press
36 Causton Street
London SW1P 4ST

Copyright © Janet Wright 2006

British Library Cataloguing-in-Publication Data
A catalogue record for this book is available from the British Library

ISBN-13: 978–0–85969–954–9
ISBN-10: 0–85969–954–4

1 3 5 7 9 10 8 6 4 2

Typeset by Deltatype Ltd, Birkenhead, Wirral
Printed in Great Britain by
Ashford Colour Press

Contents

To all those who generously
shared their information and experiences for this book,
and to David Hall, for love and support as always.

Introduction

You may have picked up this book because you have symptoms that might be early signs of the menopause, such as changes to the menstrual cycle, headaches or emotional problems. Maybe you have already started the perimenopausal transition and are seeking solutions to some of its challenges. Or you may just be wondering what the perimenopause is!

This book aims to answer all those questions, and provide information you can use in making your own decisions about this period of your life.

It can be used by women at any point in the journey towards the menopause, but it is particularly useful for women from about 35 onwards, in the early stages of hormonal change. At this age, you can take preventative measures to forestall possible problems during the years around the menopause. The action you take now can continue to affect your health and well-being into old age.

The hormonal changes that herald the perimenopause start having an impact as early as your mid-thirties. Some women may notice emotional changes, and this book explores how to deal with possible problems such as depression, mood swings, anxiety, loss of libido and insomnia. The perimenopause occurs at a busy time in most women's lives, and we could do without any needless drains on our energy. This book looks at how to have optimum health and well-being at this time so we can cope with the numerous issues we face on a daily basis. That may mean big decisions as well as smaller ones. Many women during this period are faced with the decision as to whether or not to have children. For those who decide to, this book has advice and information about improving your chances of a healthy pregnancy. For those who decide against having children, it may be time to rethink your contraceptive strategy for the next stage of your life. And for those starting a family in their late thirties or forties, this book looks at what happens when new motherhood and the perimenopause collide.

The perimenopause is a time of transition, not an illness, and most women come through it unscathed. But fluctuating hormone levels can cause a host of symptoms, some minor, some niggling, and others that can disrupt your life if left untreated. If you take the right action now, you may never have any symptoms worth worrying about.

INTRODUCTION

The advice in this book does not, however, replace medical treatment. Go to your GP if any health problems you've been treating with self-help remedies do not clear up quickly.

Don't rely on natural remedies if the symptoms could be those of a serious condition such as heart disease, diabetes or cancer – see your GP as soon as you notice them. These are things that need a correct diagnosis and medical treatment. Self-help cannot replace conventional treatment for serious illness, although it has a lot to offer alongside it.

2

1

What is the perimenopause?

The perimenopause starts in the forties for most women. But the hormonal shifts leading up to it start in the mid-thirties, when some women notice the first signs of change.

For many women, the perimenopause is so uneventful that they don't even know they've been through it till it's over. One day they tot up the length of time since their last period and realize it's been more than a year. They've sailed through the perimenopause, and the menopause itself. They may still develop a few symptoms, but these are unlikely to last long.

Not everyone is so fortunate. A few women suffer a decade or more of health problems. Luckily, the majority just get a few symptoms, which are sometimes uncomfortable or inconvenient. It's not horrific, but it can be a nuisance. And as this lasts several years, it's worth finding out how to reduce the disadvantages.

An added complication today is that people are starting families later in life, so a woman at this age may not know whether her sudden despondency is caused by baby blues or a perimenopausal mood swing.

As in so many areas, knowledge is power, so finding out what's happening is the first step to taking control of your health and well-being.

Perimenopause and menopause

The word 'perimenopause' can mean any time around menopause, including the first year or two after periods stop. But it's generally used to mean the few years between the first signs of hormonal change and the final period.

The menopause itself is just the date on which you have your last period. Because most women's cycles are irregular by that stage, this is only determined after a year with no bleeding at all.

For most women, the menopause happens in their late forties or early fifties, with the average age being 50 to 51. Anything before 40 is an early menopause, though some doctors consider up to 45 to be early. Having a hysterectomy doesn't necessarily cause the menopause, as long as you keep at least one ovary. But removal of both ovaries will cause an immediate menopause.

The perimenopause is more difficult to pin down, as it begins when you start having symptoms. That's fine if your first symptoms are clearly related to your hormones – such as changes in your menstrual cycle – but what if they're less obvious? For many women, the first signs of perimenopause were emotional or psychological – but they didn't realize what was causing these at the time. So, though we know the date when it ends, it's hard to say how long an average perimenopause lasts. The best guess, backed by research, is roughly five years. But anything up to 10 or 12 years is not uncommon.

The symptoms of the perimenopause are largely those that have usually been called 'menopausal' (see box). But your hormone levels are very different when you start the perimenopause and when you complete the menopause. So treatments that would suit a woman whose periods have nearly finished might be ineffective, or even harmful, for one who still has several years to go.

For that reason, although this book covers the entire perimenopause, it is particularly useful for women from 35 onwards, who are just starting – or are soon to start – this part of their lives.

Signs of the perimenopause

The course of a perimenopause is as individual as the woman who is going through this transition. For many women, unexpected changes in their menstrual cycle are the first definite signs of perimenopause. Periods become lighter or heavier, with flooding; or less frequent, or even totally irregular. For the first time since their teens, they'll be caught out by a sudden bleed while they're at work or out shopping. Some women also develop, for the first time in their lives, full-scale premenstrual syndrome (PMS), with aching breasts, foul temper and fluid retention. Others are startled by what seem like classic menopausal symptoms, such as hot flushes (and their after-dark manifestation, night sweats), even though their periods are still regular. In some women these are the first signs of the perimenopause, and they're also the ones that are most likely to continue for a few years after the menopause. They are called 'vasomotor' symptoms, meaning that they're caused by a sudden expansion of the blood vessels. Your temperature soars, you turn bright red, and break out in a sweat that can drench your clothes or wake you from a deep sleep.

Why this happens is mysterious. It's probably a response by the brain to a change in hormonal levels, such as a sudden drop in oestrogen. But no one yet knows why the brain should misinterpret this as a signal that body temperature has fallen.

The mental and emotional symptoms can be just as disconcerting, because the hormones that govern the reproductive system have effects far beyond the womb. Most of us have sometimes felt dejected or irritable the day before a period starts, even if we haven't encountered the violent mood swings caused by full-scale PMS. During the perimenopause, this is a reminder that these hormones affect the brain. Some women have to cope with the kind of emotional upheaval they thought they'd grown out of when they stopped reading teenage magazines. Some, on the other hand, become so distracted and forgetful that they fear they're developing Alzheimer's disease.

In fact, a surprising range of problems at this time of life are caused by the hormonal changes of the perimenopause. Some of them – such as physical clumsiness, joint pains or insomnia – seem totally unrelated to changes in the reproductive system. It's a shock when you start tripping over kerbs and breaking plates while doing the washing-up. And it's profoundly disheartening when what seem to be the aches and pains of old age appear before you even consider you've reached midlife.

It's hard to believe that all these are normal signs of changing hormonal levels, long before the end of a woman's reproductive life. Yet it's true. The big plus is that some of these symptoms are temporary and others can be reduced or reversed. Taking the right action in good time can prevent many of them becoming more serious problems as the menopause approaches.

A range of symptoms
Judith's periods had been getting heavier for some five or ten years before she started having hot flushes in her mid-forties. A fair-skinned redhead, she finds the heat overwhelming. It's a family trait, as both her sisters have similarly powerful vasomotor symptoms.

'They're the main symptoms I get, a real nuisance,' she says. 'Last Christmas when the cold weather started, my hot flushes came on along with the central heating. In the spring they eased off, but then my periods came back, which was a bore. I had three periods last year, then they came back this spring. I seem to have the hot flushes when I'm not having periods.'

Judith has tried some natural remedies such as soya milk, but suspects she isn't drinking enough of it to make a difference. 'The

Do you recognize any of these?

Perimenopausal symptoms can include:

- anxiety
- breast lumpiness
- breast pain
- clumsiness
- constipation
- depression
- dry skin
- fatigue
- fluid retention (bloating)
- forgetfulness
- heart palpitations
- heavy bleeding
- hot flushes
- insomnia
- irregular periods
- joint pains
- loss of balance
- loss of libido
- mental fuzziness
- migraine
- mood swings
- night sweats
- painful periods
- thrush
- urinary incontinence
- urinary infections
- vaginal dryness
- weight gain

Note: Many of these symptoms can be caused by other conditions. If you find a breast lump, bleed excessively, feel heart palpitations or have suicidal thoughts, see your GP at once.

trouble is, the hot flushes are sporadic,' she says. 'I don't usually know when they're going to come, so I'd have to keep taking some remedy all the time just in case. Then I wouldn't know if it had worked or I just happened not to have any hot flushes!'

Like most people she knows, she doesn't feel the symptoms are bad enough to be worth treating by going to her GP.

What's going on?

Surprisingly, for an event that almost all women go through, scientists aren't certain of the exact hormonal reasons for all the symptoms. Not so long ago, they blamed declining levels of oestrogen, and in some scientific studies blood tests seemed to back this up.

More recently, studies have shown a different hormonal picture. Women allowed researchers to take their blood several times each day, and the results were startling. They showed that levels of several reproductive hormones could vary from high to low within the space of a few hours. The proportions of different hormones in relation to each other could vary just as dramatically in the same time-frame.

The big surprise was that, far from being low in oestrogen, some women with perimenopausal symptoms had higher levels than would be expected in a young woman. They were full of oestrogen, yet they seemed to be suffering classic symptoms of oestrogen deficiency such as hot flushes and night sweats. It turned out that, though the oestrogen levels were often high, they were fluctuating wildly, and symptoms may have been caused by a sudden drop from very high levels.

What does seem to decrease steadily during this early part of the perimenopause is the production of another vital reproductive hormone, progesterone. Along with some other hormones, this works alongside oestrogen to maintain the menstrual cycle. To complicate matters, oestrogen isn't just one hormone but three: oestradiol (the strongest form), oestriol and oestrone, which all work slightly differently.

Though each hormone plays a vital role, it can be harmful in excess. Oestrogen and progesterone, in particular, work to balance each other's action so that, when everything is running smoothly, neither one causes any trouble.

For that reason, many experts believe that the most troublesome symptoms of perimenopause are caused not by a simple lack of oestrogen, but by fluctuations in oestrogen levels and by lack of progesterone to balance it. It makes sense when you think about it: if low oestrogen levels were the sole cause of perimenopausal symptoms such as hot flushes, women would be plagued with them till their dying day.

To add to the difficulties of finding out exactly what's happening, researchers believe it's not just about hormone levels. Different women may have similar test results, but with completely different symptoms, or none at all. That suggests the difference is in each brain's sensitivity to the hormones.

One theory is that the common symptoms of perimenopause, in its early stages, are caused by high or fluctuating oestrogen, and possibly follicle-stimulating hormone (FSH), or a lack of progesterone to counterbalance the oestrogen. The results are similar to those of PMS – violent mood swings, fluid retention and swollen or lumpy breasts – as well as frequent or painful periods, heavy bleeding, migraine and insomnia.

As the perimenopause continues, the body's production of oestrogen does slow down. Falling oestrogen levels then cause the classic symptoms of hot flushes and night sweats, heart palpitations and mental confusion. These happen not because oestrogen levels are necessarily low, but when they're dropping (sometimes from a high level) and the body hasn't yet adjusted. As oestrogen levels fall and stay low, you also start to notice dry skin and vaginal soreness.

Hormone levels can go on rising and falling for years, before your menstrual cycles come to an end. Even then, oestrogen production doesn't come to a total halt, but it settles at a much lower level.

After the last menstrual cycle has finished, you may go on having symptoms, especially hot flushes, for a few more years as hormone levels finally settle into their new balance. You may be startled at how much energy you regain as you get on with your life.

Forewarned is forearmed

Because the perimenopause is about fluctuating hormones, it's hard to say in advance how it is going to go. But there are clues to when it's likely to start and whether you'll get the most annoying symptoms. Some of these clues offer the chance to reduce your risk by taking action.

Take, for example, the 'vasomotor symptoms': hot flushes and night sweats. You're more likely to encounter these classic

The technical bit

Hormones are chemical messengers that relay instructions from the endocrine glands or organs where they're produced to other parts of the body. Throughout a woman's fertile life, a complex interplay of hormones works to maintain her menstrual cycle and, when possible, to facilitate a pregnancy.

At the beginning of each month – counting day 1 as the day bleeding begins – gonadotrophin-releasing hormone (GnRH) and follicle-stimulating hormone (FSH) prompt the egg follicles in the ovaries to produce oestrogen. Oestrogen levels rise until they trigger the release of luteinizing hormone (LH), which tells the ovaries to produce progesterone. The progesterone, helped by LH and FSH, then spurs one of the ovaries to release an egg. This is ovulation, which happens on about day 14 of an average 28-day cycle.

For the next eight days, the ovaries produce high levels of progesterone, which builds up the womb lining ready to nurture a fertilized egg. Progesterone and oestrogen together send a message to the brain to put production of the other hormones on hold. If a fertilized egg is implanted, it sends out a hormone that tells the ovaries to keep producing oestrogen and progesterone, so the womb lining stays in place and the next period doesn't happen. But if no egg is implanted, levels of oestrogen and progesterone start to drop, and two weeks after ovulation the womb lining breaks away and leaves the body – this is the start of the next period.

From the first day of bleeding to ovulation is called the follicular phase, and this can vary in length. From ovulation till the start of the next period, the luteal phase, is 14 days.

The perimenopause occurs when this hormonal dance begins to falter. The ovaries become less sensitive to FSH, so the body may produce more of this to stimulate the ovaries. This causes earlier ovulation, reducing the amount of time between periods. Sometimes the ovary may release a defective egg, which will generate hormones less effectively.

As the number of egg follicles decreases, you may not ovulate every month, which means there is no trigger for the ovaries to produce progesterone. Eventually this will stop your menstrual cycles, but meanwhile you may go on producing high levels of oestrogen.

perimenopausal symptoms if you have a history of PMS or irregular periods, or if you started your periods before the age of 12. Smoking and drinking seem to increase the risk, as does being either underweight or overweight. Some studies suggest that depression also increases the risk of these symptoms.

Early perimenopause may also be predicted. Smokers start one to two years earlier than average, especially if they're underweight. Yet being very overweight may also bring an early menopause. Women who have never had children may start slightly earlier too. Poor nutrition is another risk factor. One study has found that women who have experienced poverty, whether in childhood or more recently, start the perimenopause earlier. And if your periods are closer together than the standard 28-day cycle, you're likely to reach menopause sooner.

On the other hand, if you've been on the Pill for several years you may reach menopause later than average. And the more children you have, the later you're likely to stop ovulating. But you can't delay the menopause by stopping your periods, as it's not just a question of conserving eggs. Women whose periods have stopped for less healthy reasons, such as being severely underweight, are likely to reach the menopause earlier.

Anything that damages the ovaries can bring the perimenopause forward. This can be the result of medical treatments such as radiotherapy or of autoimmune diseases such as rheumatoid arthritis. After a hysterectomy, the ovaries may not function so well. (If both your ovaries are removed too, you will have an immediate menopause.)

There's a definite genetic link too: if your mother or other relatives had an early menopause, you're likely to follow suit. Even your birthday may have an effect: Italian research claims that women reach the menopause two years earlier if they were born in spring than those born in autumn!

If you're noticing perimenopausal signs before the age of 40, your GP may do a test for the reproductive hormone FSH, which increases as your ovary function winds down. High levels of FSH are a sign that you have started the perimenopause. You may also have your oestrogen levels tested, but this can be misleading as they fluctuate dramatically and may even be high during the early stages of perimenopause.

In the near future, researchers hope it will be possible to check the number of eggs remaining in a woman's ovaries with an ultrasound scan, though this won't reveal how healthy the eggs are. Other researchers are working on drugs that will slow down the rate at which the ovaries lose eggs.

Perimenopause and the Pill

How do you know you've reached the perimenopause if you're on the Pill? When you've found a Pill that works for you, you have no heavy bleeding. Your 'periods' are perfectly regular because they're just breakthrough bleeds during the week you don't take a Pill.

The combined oestrogen and progestogen Pill has been found to reduce or prevent hot flushes and night sweats. You may start to notice some of the other symptoms, such as anxiety or mood swings, but many women never suffer from these, whether they're on the Pill or not. So you may not know when the perimenopause starts, or even when you have gone through the menopause.

Though it's not important at this stage, it matters when you pass the menopause. The hormones you're taking in the Pill are too high for your body's needs after you've naturally stopped ovulating, and could increase your risk of cancer. You should ask your GP or well-woman clinic about having tests if you're still on the Pill at 50, or if you have any reason to think that menopause has occurred before then.

If you smoke, or if you have any health-risk factors that make the combined Pill unsuitable after the age of 35, you may be on the progestogen-only Pill. This is less likely to mask signs of the perimenopause, so although you won't have irregular periods you may notice some of the other symptoms, such as hot flushes.

You can also have FSH and oestrogen tests, although the results aren't 100 per cent accurate. These tests should be done on the last Pill-free day of your cycle.

Reducing the risk of cancer

Some cancers, especially those of the uterus (womb) and breast, are strongly affected by our reproductive hormones, particularly oestrogen. Though cancer becomes much more common after 50, women in their thirties are at risk of developing the most invasive forms, which grow and spread rapidly, fuelled by an abundant supply of oestrogen.

After the menopause, this risk is reduced. But during the perimenopause, it may be higher than before. As progesterone levels fall, the body's production of oestrogen continues unabated for a while, and during this time oestrogen levels may be higher than ever.

Because levels of these hormones may wax and wane within a few hours, it's difficult to take accurate readings even if you're having your hormone levels tested.

Heavy bleeding can be a sign of very high oestrogen levels, but you can still have high oestrogen levels without bleeding heavily. If other women in your family have had these cancers, you are at higher risk. Breast and ovarian cancers tend to run in the same family, as do cancers of the bowel and endometrium. There's even a possibility that all four may run in the same family. So if you had a grandparent or uncle who died of, say, bowel cancer, you're at higher risk of endometrial cancer and possibly of breast or ovarian cancer. Heavy bleeding could indicate a problem with your endometrium, so don't delay in seeing your doctor and telling him or her about the family history of bowel cancer.

The genetic link isn't the only risk factor, though, so if any unusual symptom lasts for more than a few days, get your GP to check it out.

External influences

Hormone function can be affected by pollution from chemicals we're in contact with every day, known as xenoestrogens, or endocrine disrupters. We encounter them as residues on food, dry-cleaning fumes, herbicides in green spaces and numerous other forms. These are among a wide range of chemicals known to disrupt hormone functions in animals. Initially mimicking the effects of oestrogen, they then confuse the animal's hormone system into producing deformed offspring, becoming infertile, developing cancer or even changing from male to female.

The effects on human beings are less well tested, but they have been linked with breast and other cancers. Endocrine disrupters found in pesticides, detergents and even food wrap have been shown to increase the division rate of breast-cancer cells in test tubes. And though the evidence is disputed by some authorities, it looks as if they have caused cancer in human beings.

It's not yet known whether they affect our bodily processes in other ways. But, as they behave in some ways like oestrogen, there is at least a possibility that they could exacerbate the perimenopausal symptoms linked with fluctuating oestrogen levels. They may also reduce fertility and increase the risk of miscarriage.

To reduce your risk from various possibly hormone-disrupting chemicals

- Use heat-resistant glass containers in the microwave instead of plastic.
- Store fatty foods such as cheese in airtight glass or china containers instead of cling film.
- Buy organic fruit and vegetables where possible. You still need to wash them, but only to remove surface dirt instead of scrubbing off chemical residues – many of which permeate the produce anyway.
- Try to buy only organic meat and dairy products. If you can't buy organic, cut down on fatty meat, as many chemicals are stored in fat.
- Drink from glass or china, not from plastic or disposable cups. If you buy a bottle of water to drink, don't keep refilling the bottle afterwards: buy a water bottle from a camping shop to fill and carry with you, as the bottles sold with drinks in them aren't made for reusing.
- Don't use organophosphate pesticides on pets or gardens (or anywhere else).
- Look for a dry-cleaner who uses water-based solvents – or, better still, save a lot of money and buy clothes that don't need dry-cleaning! If you're bringing dry-cleaning home in the car, leave the windows open because the fumes build up in an enclosed space.
- Buy unbleached paper, made without chlorine.
- Try to avoid vinyl and PVC.
- Use the gentlest, environment-friendly household cleaners you can find.
- If you play golf, don't touch your face after picking up the ball, and keep away from the course when it's recently been sprayed. Most golf courses are sprayed intensively.

Puberty in reverse?

The perimenopause has been called 'puberty in reverse' – think unpredictable periods, mood swings and problems with your skin! You were leaving childhood behind and embarking on a journey into

13

an unknown new role. And for every woman with happy memories of her fun-packed teens, there's another who wouldn't return to that tumultuous time for anything.

But one big difference is that, back then, you had very little experience of the world, and few resources for dealing with change. You'd never had any responsibilities before; you were being pushed on to what looked like an endless conveyor belt of things you had to do, with very little control over your own life.

This time around, you have two to three extra decades of life experience, more realistic expectations, and enough knowledge to find the resources you need. You have lifelong friends who won't drop you after a squabble. And though the information in this book should help you have an easier transition than you did in your teens, you don't have to memorize it for an exam!

2
Could it be something else?

If you're 45 and getting the classic hot flushes and irregular periods, you're likely to have entered the perimenopause. But what if you're 36 and your periods have become heavy and frequent? Or at 42 you're suffering from heart palpitations and unexplained fatigue? Or you're 39, getting thicker round the middle and aching in the joints, but your periods are still regular and you've had no other signs of change?

Those could also be perimenopausal symptoms, but they're just as likely to have other causes. Many of the other conditions that cause perimenopause-like effects are quite harmless, and can be easily treated, so it's worth having a correct diagnosis and not just putting up with them.

But some of these symptoms can also be caused by serious conditions that need immediate treatment. Don't run the risk if you have any of these: go to your GP at once. You shouldn't accept any symptom, especially pain, without finding out the cause, and what you can do about it.

If your symptoms do prove to be perimenopause, see the chapters on self-help and alternative remedies, and what your GP can do for you.

It may not be your time of life
Lucy, 46, wondered if her tiredness, tension and heart palpitations could be signs of perimenopause. Her periods were becoming lighter and she never felt quite well any more. She was finding it increasingly difficult to cope with problems: when water poured through her ceiling – as it frequently did – she could hardly breathe as she banged on the door of the upstairs flat.

The day her heart fluttered so violently that she briefly lost consciousness, she decided to seek help. To her surprise, her GP sent her to a cardiologist. The specialist ran a series of tests, and found that Lucy's coronary arteries were so blocked that she could have a heart attack at any moment.

'I can't have heart disease at my age,' she wailed. 'I don't even smoke!' The doctor admitted it was hard to say what had caused it, as she was only slightly overweight and had no family history of early heart problems. Years of stress must have taken their toll.

An earlier illness may have damaged the coronary arteries, and perhaps her diet was less healthy than she liked to think. The cause wasn't obvious, but the cure was. A coronary bypass took her off the danger list, and after that she made some healthy changes to her lifestyle.

Since then, she says, she has heard of many women who turned out to have serious diseases after being told their symptoms were harmless signs of hormonal change.

'My GP saved my life, but I was lucky,' she says. 'Don't accept that everything that happens in your forties is about the perimenopause. If you feel there's something wrong, go to your GP. If you're told it's just your age, or just stress, ask for tests to rule out anything else. Or find another doctor!'

Menstrual symptoms

Heavy bleeding often happens early in the perimenopause, when progesterone levels are falling. Progesterone helps the womb shed its lining, and without enough progesterone the lining may continue to grow, causing a much heavier bleed when it does come away. But if you're losing a lot more blood than usual, there may be something else at work. Does your period usually start less than three weeks after the start of the last one? Does it last more than six days? Do you soak through a pad or tampon within a couple of hours, or have to change them during the night? Do you lose spots of blood between periods, or after love-making?

Heavy bleeding can also be a sign of growths such as fibroids, which develop in the wall of the womb, or polyps, which develop in the cervix (the neck of the womb) or the womb lining. They're not dangerous in themselves, and don't lead to cancer. But they can cause other symptoms, including pain, especially during sex or during periods, and may make you more likely to miscarry. It could be a sign of endometriosis – in which tissue from the lining of the womb grows in other parts of the abdomen – which can spread, causing chronic pain and infertility. It could even mean your thyroid gland isn't working properly, which can be treated.

Occasionally, heavy or frequent bleeding can be caused by certain cancers, or by endometrial hyperplasia – an excessive growth of the womb lining, which can develop into cancer. So, see your GP if you're bleeding more often or more heavily than in the past. A cancer needs immediate treatment, and then has a high success rate.

Even if the cause is harmless, constant heavy bleeding can cause exhaustion and iron-deficiency anaemia.

Premenstrual syndrome

Mood swings, depression, irritability, fluid retention, swollen breasts – PMS or perimenopause? Just to confuse matters, women often do develop PMS during the perimenopause, especially in the first stage. There are some clues to help you differentiate between PMS and perimenopause, though they're not foolproof.

PMS usually strikes during the second half of your cycle and is relieved by the start of a period. The difference between the night before and the morning your period starts can be quite dramatic. When the same symptoms are caused by perimenopause, they may last throughout a menstrual cycle or appear at any stage. They don't usually disappear when your period begins.

Vasomotor symptoms

Even hot flushes can have causes other than the perimenopause. An overactive thyroid is one culprit; less often, certain cancers. They can happen as a side effect of drugs prescribed for anxiety, depression, cancer or high blood pressure.

A mild flush can be triggered by heat, stress, spicy food, alcohol or coffee. Some skin conditions, such as rosacea, have a reddening effect. If you're suffering night sweats without also getting flushes during the day, you're probably just getting too hot in bed. But if it feels as if someone has suddenly thrown a bucket of hot water in your face, and you're not taking any drug known to cause this, you're probably experiencing the hormonal changes of the perimenopause.

If this seems unlikely – especially if you're young and have no other symptoms, as hot flushes often come towards the end of the perimenopause – see your GP.

Urinary and vaginal symptoms

As levels of reproductive hormones decline, most women notice that their vagina feels drier. Oestrogen keeps the walls of the vagina and urethra firm and healthy, so as oestrogen levels drop, the walls become thinner and more easily damaged.

This can make intercourse painful, leading to soreness and promoting infections such as thrush: a yeasty discharge that itches and has an unpleasant smell. Similarly, the urethra becomes more prone to infections such as cystitis, in which urination is difficult and painful. Consult your pharmacist or GP.

If you see blood in your urine, though, visit your GP without delay. This could mean a bladder infection, which, though usually simple to cure, needs immediate treatment.

Other effects of the weakened urethra walls are stress incontinence and urinary urgency. Urinary incontinence can also have other causes, such as a prolapsed womb, which can be surgically corrected.

Kegel exercises (see Chapter 7), to strengthen the pelvic floor, may take six weeks or more to show an effect. If you don't notice an improvement within a few weeks, go to your well-woman clinic or ask your GP for a referral to a specialist. Vaginal soreness, discharge or itchiness can also be an early sign of diabetes, especially if you're overweight. If you are also tired and find you're constantly thirsty and wanting to urinate, again consult your GP without delay. Diabetes is on the increase, but can be controlled.

Infections and discharges can be signs of sexually transmitted diseases (STDs). The specialist staff at genitourinary medicine (GUM) clinics are helpful and perfectly used to seeing people of all types and ages. Most STDs are straightforward to treat, but if left untreated can cause a lot of internal damage – and, of course, will be passed on to your partner.

Urinary incontinence and vaginal soreness don't usually mean anything more sinister than lack of oestrogen. See the chapters on self-help and medical treatments for what to do. If they become a real problem, visit your well-woman clinic or ask your GP for a referral to a specialist.

Weight gain and skin changes

These are two things that most women notice during this period. Sad to say, unlike many other signs of the perimenopause, they won't wear off by themselves and there's nothing you can take for them!

Skin ageing is a fact of life, though you can reduce its effects with the right kind of food and exercise as well as with creams. As for weight gain, your metabolism naturally slows down during your forties, so you just need less fuel. (See the chapters on eating and exercise for easy ways to stay at a healthy weight and keep your skin looking its best.)

But when both weight gain and skin changes coincide, and don't seem to fit the normal pattern, they could be caused by certain health conditions:

Polycystic ovarian syndrome is when cysts grow inside the ovaries, causing a number of symptoms such as acne, weight gain (especially around the middle), irregular periods or hair growth on the face and body. It's a hormonal malfunction that increases production of the 'male' hormones, androgens, among other effects, and can lead to infertility. Sometimes taking the contraceptive Pill is enough to solve the problem; otherwise, doctors have other drugs they can prescribe. If you're overweight, slimming down a bit can also help.

An underactive thyroid gland will also affect your skin, making it cold and dry, even scaly. You're likely to put on weight, while feeling lethargic and depressed. Many of the symptoms, such as muscle pains and constipation, could be taken for those of the perimenopause – your periods may even stop. But if the exhaustion is serious enough to affect your life, especially if your hair is brittle or your voice becomes hoarse, go to your GP. If you're not producing enough thyroid hormone, your GP can do a simple test for thyroid-stimulating hormone (TSH), and prescribe thyroxine if necessary.

Change of shape

Whether or not you put on much weight, you're likely to notice your waist becoming thicker towards the end of the perimenopause. As your oestrogen levels fall, weight tends to settle on your stomach and abdomen instead of your hips and thighs as before.

But if you notice this before any other signs of changing hormone levels, take a good look in a mirror. If you see any other changes, such as round shoulders or a thickening at the back of your neck, you might be seeing the first signs of the brittle-bone condition called osteoporosis.

Alarm bells should ring if you also suffer from backache or painful bones or joints. These can be harmless signs of perimeno-pause, but in conjunction with your changing shape they suggest that you might be starting to get tiny cracks in your spine.

Osteoporosis doesn't just affect older women. You're at risk if you've ever been on stringent low-calorie diets, suffered from eating disorders, over-exercised or become very thin for any other reason. Another clue is if you've ever stopped having periods for more than a couple of months when you weren't pregnant.

There are drugs you can take to reduce the rate of bone loss, but prevention is by far the best cure for osteoporosis. See your GP if it's already happening, and see the later chapters in this book for advice on eating and exercising.

Joint or muscle pain

These are perimenopausal symptoms that most of us don't expect. They can, of course, also have other causes, such as injury, overuse or arthritis.

At an age when you've been working for about 20 years and have probably become less fit than when you started, you may be feeling the results of unsuitable work equipment or bad postural habits. If you use a keyboard, you may be experiencing repetitive strain injury. Do try and remain active, and consult your GP about possible referral to a physiotherapist.

Migraine

Fluctuating levels of oestrogen cause some women to get their first-ever migraines during the perimenopause. This severe headache often affects just one side of the head; you may feel sick and find that light hurts your eyes. It's not much comfort, when you've crawled back to bed with the curtains tightly shut, to know that the menopause should put an end to your migraines. However, again, don't just put up with it. Consult your pharmacist or GP about pain relief.

Severe headaches can be caused by all kinds of health conditions, including high blood pressure. Again, see your GP if your headaches worry you for any reason. They can also be caused by normal midlife changes in your eyesight, so have your eyes checked by an optometrist to see if you need glasses or contact lenses.

Backache

A common problem as you approach your forties, backache usually has simple causes – such as poor posture, wearing high heels, spending too much time on your feet, or sleeping on a worn-out mattress. It's easy to treat with self-help or complementary therapies.

But lower back pain can sometimes stem from gynaecological problems, and it is worth having this checked if sensible lifestyle changes don't help. Backache is, occasionally, the first warning of a growth on one of the internal organs.

Unexplained exhaustion

Tiredness by itself isn't necessarily a symptom of anything except women's endlessly hectic lives. If you're going out to work, running a home, bringing up a family, and trying to keep a fragment of social life, it's not surprising if you feel worn out. Or you could just be trying to survive on too little sleep.

There may be specific culprits, however. Medication can cause daytime drowsiness, including sleeping pills, codeine and antihist-amines (found in some remedies for colds, allergies and travel sickness), so look out for warnings on the packet. Stimulants of any kind, even caffeine, can also disrupt normal sleep patterns.

But what if the exhaustion is permanent, or settles on you at odd times when you can't see any reason for it? Don't just put up with it. Fatigue can be a symptom of the perimenopause, but it can also be a sign of numerous health conditions, some of them serious.

It could be an undiagnosed sleep disorder, such as sleep apnoea (or its milder version, hypopnea) in which your throat closes while you're unconscious, stopping you breathing properly and causing shallow, unrefreshing sleep. It's more likely if you're overweight, especially around the neck. Sleep apnoea can be dangerous if left untreated, so you may be offered a sleep mask to keep the airway open. If that doesn't work, an operation should solve the problem.

If you sometimes feel breathless or dizzy, it might be heart disease, especially if you smoke. If your skin is very dry and you're putting on weight, your thyroid gland may have become underactive. If you've never quite got back on your feet after a viral infection, it could be ME (myalgic encephalomyelitis, sometimes known as chronic fatigue syndrome). If you're constantly thirsty, it could be diabetes. If you're pale and your mouth is sore, it could be anaemia. The list goes on . . .

Don't hazard a guess! Make a list of your symptoms, visit your GP and get a diagnosis. *Always* see your doctor to check out any unusual symptoms, especially those that could mean a serious condition.

3
Emotional disturbances

Mood swings and emotional upheaval are often the earliest signs of the perimenopause, including depression, anxiety and loss of libido, linked with an increasing incidence of premenstrual syndrome (PMS) at this time. Normally good-natured women suddenly find themselves yelling like an irate character in a TV soap over some minor disagreement – and an hour later wondering what all the fuss was about. Many women feel vaguely anxious without being able to say what's worrying them. Others may also find themselves forgetting people's names or losing everything they put down, and may wonder if these are early signs of Alzheimer's.

These are not the sort of thing you associate with reproductive hormones, but they *are* behind all these events. A sudden drop in oestrogen, for example, is believed to trigger the production of stress hormones such as cortisol, making you feel anxious and jittery for no apparent reason. In other words: no, you're not losing your mind! Anxiety, depression and mental fuzziness are the results of changes in hormone levels.

The good news is that much of this will settle down by itself after the menopause: women over 50 are statistically much less likely to be unhappy than those 10 or 15 years younger. But that leaves a long time to grit your teeth and endure emotional symptoms that, in many cases, can be alleviated.

It's not surprising that so many women suffer depression as they approach the menopause. We live in a society that prizes youth and sexual prowess, with the warning that after 35 it's all downhill. We see few images of older women, and most of those are negative. In your thirties and early forties you're still young – you're not expecting trouble with your hormones. Realizing that you've started a process leading to the menopause is depressing in itself, as psychologists have found.

Encouragingly, researchers have found that perimenopausal women actually score as well as younger women in brain and memory tests, even if they thought they were becoming forgetful. Only those who suffered from menopausal mood swings did less well in the tests, confirming that it's a hormonal problem – and temporary.

There are other, more complex links with psychological changes too. Women who have troublesome vasomotor symptoms (hot flushes and night sweats) are more likely to suffer from depression during the perimenopause. Not surprising, you may say, if you've ever struggled through a work meeting or school parents' day while mopping sweat from your face and neck. But it's not just that the symptoms bring these women down. Other disruptive symptoms don't necessarily lead to depression.

Doctors suspect that long-term depression dampens the body's production of hormones. That does seem likely: depression is already known to cause physical damage, increasing the risk of numerous conditions including heart disease and probably cancer. It reduces the body's ability to recover from illness and increases the risk of premature death – not only from suicide, but from apparently unrelated diseases.

Researchers studying this effect have linked it with stress, pointing out that disturbing events – and especially long-term stress – can cause depression, anxiety and physical ill health. Depression, in turn, can cause anxiety, and put physical stress on the body.

Long-term stress and depression seem to bring an earlier menopause too, especially in women who have taken antidepressants. One study found that women who had their final period before the age of 47 were three times more likely than average to have a history of depression. And women who already suffered from depression have been found to suffer more severe vasomotor symptoms.

So the psychological and emotional symptoms of perimenopause are at least partly caused by hormonal changes. But as the research shows, it's a two-way street: our emotional states have a strong influence on hormone production too. This means that a vicious circle can easily develop, in which hormonal disruption increases feelings of anxiety and depression, which in turn put stress on the body, making hormonal levels fluctuate ever more unhealthily.

'Don't mess with me!'

Although hormones are known to affect our emotions, it's less widely recognized that it works the other way round too. Hertha was in her forties when her periods suddenly stopped for three months. 'I was at exploding point the whole time and desperately tired with it,' she says. 'That's when I was winding up my divorce, which was no more pleasant than most divorces.'

Her periods returned, but her old obliging nature was never quite the same. 'I stopped being such a dishcloth,' she says.

Hertha sees a link between the jolt in her menstrual cycle and in her outlook. She has noted similar changes in friends who are also going through the perimenopause. 'We're much less willing to take nonsense, and much more assertive,' she says. 'I haven't had many other symptoms – such heat waves as have struck are barely worth mentioning. What I have had was quite an emotional change, as in "Don't mess with me!" And if you're used to messing with me, you'll have a surprise!'

For Hertha the changes have mainly been positive, but she started a new relationship after the divorce and has had a lot of emotional support from her new partner. 'I dread to think how I would have felt had I not divorced,' she adds.

Options for treatment

One solution offered by psychiatrists and many GPs is antidepressants. Tranquillizers and older forms of antidepressants were shown to cause serious side effects, but the more recent selective serotonin-reuptake inhibitors (SSRIs) were heralded as a harmless and helpful solution. The most famous of these, Prozac (fluoxetine), was even considered as a lifestyle drug for healthy people, improving their self-confidence and enjoyment of life.

Once again, however, reports of serious side effects have knocked the SSRIs off their pedestal. They have been linked with unexpected suicide and uncharacteristic violence. SSRIs are no longer prescribed to teenagers in Britain, and are given to adults with strong warnings.

In low doses, though, SSRIs have been found to relieve both perimenopausal depression and vasomotor symptoms in some women. If you are badly troubled by these symptoms and self-help measures haven't helped, SSRIs may be worth trying. Many people benefit from them without noticing any bothersome effects. Possible side effects include sleep disturbances, nausea, loss of libido and constipation or diarrhoea. But even these may be more tolerable than endless hot flushes or feeling totally out of control. You need to take the drugs regularly as prescribed, and it may take a few weeks before you notice the benefits.

Note: The risk of suicide or violence is small, but important. If you're taking SSRIs, you need to stay very aware of your feelings and reactions, and return to your GP at once if you start going downhill. The risks seem to be greatest both when you've just started taking the drug, and again if you stop taking it abruptly. If you do experience side effects, don't come off SSRIs without letting your doctor know and reducing the dose gradually as instructed.

The talking cure

Psychotherapy or counselling seems like a constructive way of dealing with depression, anxiety and other mood disorders; unlike drugs, it offers the chance to solve the problem itself rather than just damping down the symptoms for a while. But recent research suggests that psychotherapy offers more than it can deliver. Several studies have shown that people who have long-term psychotherapy end up no happier or better-balanced than people in similar circumstances who didn't have therapy. It may even be harmful: some studies have shown that people are more depressed and find it harder to cope with their problems after counselling than before.

Some forms are less helpful than others. Traditional psychoanalysis continues for years, keeping the patient dependent on the person who is supposedly helping them. Psychoanalysts do at least have to be qualified, but other psychotherapists don't have to be – they may have years of training or none at all. Digging up childhood experiences can bring to light all kinds of trauma, which an inexperienced therapist may not know how to handle, leaving the client in a worse state than before.

Hypnotherapy offers a short-cut to the sub-conscious mind, with brilliant results in the right circumstances. But it has been known to bring up demons that the client can't cope with, or even implant ideas about events that never happened. In experiments, volunteers who are hypnotized don't necessarily recall events more clearly than without hypnosis – but they are more convinced that their recollections are accurate.

One form of psychotherapy that regularly proves its worth in research studies is cognitive behavioural therapy, or CBT. This very successful short form of therapy focuses on the present rather than the past. It aims to help people solve the problems they have now, instead of delving into long-ago grievances. It does this by helping clients to discover what they're doing that's holding them back and to change the outlook that underpins these counter-productive behaviour patterns. Various schools of thought have produced a number of variations on CBT, with names such as rational emotive therapy. With slightly different outlooks and techniques, they all aim to help people move on from where they're stuck.

A course of CBT runs for a pre-arranged number of sessions, with both you and the therapist aiming to reach a satisfactory conclusion by the final appointment. If you haven't solved every problem, you should at least be able to cope with those that have been causing you most grief.

'I'd rather go to sleep...'

Loss of sex drive is not necessarily always a problem: if you're contentedly single, you may simply put your energy to other uses. But you may find the loss of such a familiar pleasure hard to accept, or it may put a strain on a relationship that has included sex up till now. Some researchers have found that men, on average, want to make love about twice as frequently as women.

The cause for a loss of libido can be as simple as sheer exhaustion, especially if, like many women, you started a family in your thirties and are now coping with small children. In this case, try to off-load some of your responsibilities, and get your children doing some of their own chores. Try to take occasional nights away with your partner – for your health as much as for your sex life. Don't be reluctant about appealing for help with childcare from friends and relatives: the kids can enjoy a weekend with their cousins or grandparents while you and your partner enjoy each other.

Routine is another factor. There's no denying that the magic can go out of even the best marriage after 15 years, two kids and several thousand kisses. Books, DVDs and your own imagination can help, backed up by willingness and a sense of humour.

Loss of libido is part of the energy-sapping effects of many diseases, and could be an early sign of something going wrong. It is also a side effect of many drugs, including the progesterone-only contraceptive pill. It's not always stated as a side effect, so if you notice a change when you've been taking any medicine, look it up online or ask your GP. Don't stop taking any necessary medicine without consulting your doctor, who may be able to adjust the dose or prescribe a more suitable drug.

Depression frequently reduces people's interest in sex, along with other sources of pleasure. But be careful in treating it, as loss of libido is a common side effect of antidepressants too. However, treatments that help you regain your pleasure in life more naturally could bring your libido back as well.

Hormonal changes can also reduce libido, and these may begin insidiously before you were expecting them. Many women find their skin becomes increasingly sensitive to discomfort, while vaginal dryness may cause irritation or pain.

Hormone replacement therapy (HRT) can bring back a lost libido and restore vaginal lubrication; some women find that phytoestrogen alternatives help. For skin that's become over-sensitive, you may find that lighter or firmer pressure helps, and perhaps learning massage techniques.

Oils or moisturizers, or vaginal lubricants, also help some women. Don't just use the first lubricant you try, as there are very different formulations available in a range of applicators. You need enough lubrication to feel comfortable but without deadening all sensation, so a thick gel may be more than you need.

Building emotional resilience

Depression and anxiety are strongly influenced, in most people, by circumstances as well as hormones. During the perimenopause, doctors have found that women are more likely to become depressed if they sleep badly (quite apart from the fact that depression can cause insomnia), and less likely if they are in paid employment. Divorce, bereavement and job loss are other obvious factors contributing to depression. Some of the events that predispose people to anxiety or depression cast their shadow from the past, and a *good* therapist (see comments earlier) can help a client to exorcize these ghosts.

But resilience seems to be a life skill that can be learned. Psychologists have noted that some people deal more successfully than others with what life throws at them. In fact, they seem to sail blithely through events that would drive anyone else to drink. Researchers have found that people who seem immune to anxiety or depression, no matter what their backgrounds, all tend to have a similar set of attitudes and coping strategies. The recommendations in this chapter are based on numerous studies of emotional resilience. We need to accept our limitations and stop berating ourselves for not creating a perfect life. We need to let go of any perfectionist tendencies. The more we try to keep control of every detail, the higher the chances are that we'll be disappointed in at least one area. Perfectionism also puts the people around us under pressure to meet our standards. They may either refuse to do this, which offends us, or make efforts that they secretly resent. All are

27

recipes for dissatisfaction and conflict. If we can't change the situation, say the experts, we need to change the way we view it. That doesn't necessarily mean spending a lot of time poring over what's gone wrong. Some researchers have found that people who push upsetting thoughts out of their minds are happier and more successful. Those who are more aware of their feelings often tend to be less happy or satisfied. This may be why long-term psychotherapy has such low rates of success – whatever the other benefits of self-examination, it doesn't seem to make people happier or more confident.

People who spend a lot of time brooding over their problems have also been found to have a lower opinion of themselves. This is significant because self-esteem is one of the most important elements of mental health: people who believe in themselves are much less likely to be thrown into perimenopausal doubt or self-hate when they forget a relative's name or have a hot flush during a meeting at work.

Letting go of perfectionism has an added benefit. Easy-going people don't just shake off doubts and disasters more easily – their personalities make them less likely to engage in conflict of any kind. And though conflict makes good television, it makes a very dismal reality. Soap operas may thrive on furious arguments followed by passionate reconciliations, but in the real world the arguments become steadily more bitter and the reconciliations less sincere.

A lot of research has overturned the idea that getting things off your chest is necessarily better than bottling them up. That hormone-fuelled explosion isn't just embarrassing – it could double our risk of a heart attack. Researchers emphasize that it is specifically expressing hostility rather than just feeling it that causes the damage. Bouts of anger simply increase our stress levels rather than relieving them.

Not that we should keep genuine grievances simmering under a lid. Psychologists recommend either talking things through with the person who annoyed us (expressing anger if necessary) or solving the problem as best we can, then getting on with our lives. Try doing relaxation techniques such as breathing exercises to soothe yourself when you feel the irritation rising.

Taking responsibility for ourselves is an important part of maintaining self-esteem during the perimenopause. If we accept commitments, we don't feel trapped by them. No matter what life (or our terrible toddler) throws at us, self-pity is the worst response. Seeing ourselves as victims stops us taking control of our lives and promotes the feelings of helplessness that cause despair. Studies of happy and well-balanced people show that they see setbacks as challenges and face up to them. This doesn't necessarily distract them from their personal goals. They are clear about what these are, and they work towards them.

Maintaining close ties with family and friends helps us to stay on top of events, but it's important for these relationships to be supportive and positive. Having supportive friends can also help us to cope with difficult family relationships. During the often confusing changes of the perimenopause, this support is more important than ever.

Happy and successful people live balanced lives with time for exercise and relaxation. Exercise helps us to cope with emotional upheaval and encourages the body to produce feel-good hormones such as serotonin, a vital pick-me-up when we're feeling stressed or unhappy. But it has to be exercise for fun. If we've a tendency to become highly competitive or self-critical, then we shouldn't take up a sport or pursuit that will fuel this drive.

'You're never prepared for how it feels'

For Moira, a careers adviser, the perimenopause is a time of questioning and assessment. 'I feel as if I've gone straight from teens to old age without adulthood,' she says. 'I haven't got used to being a mature person and suddenly I'm old, and where did my adult life go?'

Changing hormone levels have affected her emotionally more than physically, she finds. Always even-tempered in the past, she is now a lot less tolerant. 'I find myself getting furious at times, in a way I never did before,' she says. 'I used to be more patient and tolerant. It was never an effort, it just came naturally.'

In her late forties, her periods have become irregular and unpredictable, but she is happy for them to continue. 'I like that evidence of womanhood every month. It's a lifelong companion that you're going to lose, whatever you feel about them.'

Having lost both parents, and with a family history of high blood pressure and heart disease, Moira has had to give up her insouciant outlook and take a more protective attitude towards her health. Though she's tall, slim and fit, the fact that her hair started greying early has had an effect too. 'I've got into paler colours, like lavender,' she says. 'I'd never have thought of wearing lavender before! But bright colours now make my hair look as if it's faded. So I'm toning down the colours. It's all adjusting, a rite of passage.

'I watched a programme about women approaching the

menopause, and they all said the same thing – they felt as if they had become invisible. I don't feel invisible yet, but I wonder if it's going to happen. A month ago a young woman stood up for me on the bus and gave me her seat. Instead of being grateful, I felt furious! A whole shockwave went through me: this is going to happen from now on. I'm going to be seen as someone who might possibly be frail. Being referred to as "the lady" and "madam".

'However much you know what's going to happen, I don't think you're ever prepared for how it feels.'

Regaining control

- Make a point of controlling your temper if you lose it easily: it really does get easier with practice. Try simple tactics like counting to ten or walking away.
- Look for the opportunities in things that happen to you. For example, a missed train can be an opportunity to spend time alone having a quiet sit-down with a coffee.
- Stay close to friends and family and spend time with them.
- Work out your personal goals and check that you're on course towards them.
- If you're always late and flustered, get some help with time-management skills.
- Share a whinge session with friends when you need to, then drop the subject.
- Try cognitive behaviour therapy if you feel stuck.
- Healthy eating, relaxation and regular exercise all help to maintain your equilibrium.

4

Contraception and fertility

During their late thirties many women find themselves facing the decision they've been putting off for years: do they want to have children? Because, if so, it's time to do something about it. After 20 years of being careful about contraception, you may be delighted to drop your Pills in the bin and stop off at Mothercare on the way home from work. But don't risk disappointment by expecting to fall pregnant the first night. Conception at this age may take longer than expected.

Throughout your twenties you have a 1-in-4 chance of conceiving each time you make love at the right time of the month. That's around the time of ovulation – about 14 days before your next period is due. Fertility starts dropping off in your late twenties to early thirties, but until your mid-thirties, the chance is still 1-in-6. This declines in your late thirties. The average 40-year-old woman has a 1-in-10 chance, and by 45 this is down to a 1-in-25 chance. Our bodies age at different rates, partly for genetic reasons and partly as a result of how well we've looked after ourselves. But these figures show that, by 40, even a healthy woman will take much longer to conceive than she would have done ten years earlier. She is also likely to have an older partner, whose sperm may be less active.

Think about it

Are you sure you want a baby now? Or do you think you have to seize the chance before it disappears? Are you starting to feel left out as the last few of your childless friends become pregnant? Are you under pressure from everyone who insists that you'll be happier if you have children?

If so, weigh up the options. If you have a child in your mid to late thirties, you'll be going through the menopause just as he or she reaches puberty – next stop, hormone hell. If you're over 40, you may be thinking wistfully about retirement while you're working overtime to pay for university fees. As grown-up children now often stay at home into their late twenties or even thirties, you may be doing their laundry until the day you move into a retirement village. And your longed-for grandchildren may arrive too late for you to enjoy them.

Bear in mind that, statistically, pregnancy is riskier in your late thirties or forties. The chances are that all will go well, but miscarriage, ectopic pregnancy (when the fertilized egg starts growing outside the womb) or a baby with a congenital condition are possible realities. Medical tests can check for some conditions, but are not foolproof; also, they can cause the miscarriage of a healthy baby. And of course if the test reveals a possible health problem, you are then faced with the painful decision of whether to end the pregnancy.

Don't feel you're out on a limb in a world full of parents. Though only 1 in 11 60-year-old women is childless, that is a historically low number. Among women now approaching the menopause, 1 in 5 is expected to have no children – about the same as in earlier generations. And surveys often find that childless couples are happier than those who have had children, even if their childlessness was not intentional.

'I've never felt adult'

'I wonder if it's because of not having children that I've never really felt adult?' says Moira, who lives with her partner of 20 years.

'I'm starting to accept that I'll never have children now, and wondering if I should have done. Because I'm gay, I come to it from a different perspective, because it would be such an effort to get pregnant. But from being an intellectual question, it's become something much more emotional now.'

Contraceptive options

If you don't want to become pregnant, this is a good time to reconsider your contraceptive options.

Up till the age of 35, the combined Pill, containing both oestrogen and progestogen, is a popular form of contraception. You can stay on it till the menopause, according to current health advice, as long as you're in a low-risk group.

You may find the combined Pill helpful in perimenopause as it prevents heavy bleeding and the problems of exhaustion and anaemia. Because the Pill stops you ovulating, there's very little womb lining to shed during the monthly bleed.

It has also been found to solve other perimenopausal problems, including hot flushes. Some women go further and say it wipes out all the symptoms, from anxiety to breast lumps. It replaces your fluctuating hormones with a constant dose of oestrogen and progestogen, especially if you take a monophasic Pill such as Loestrin, Microgynon or Cileste. These deliver the same amount of oestrogen and progestogen every day. Triphasic Pills such as Logynon vary the formulation at different times of the month.

Like HRT, the Pill comes in numerous different strengths and formulations, and it may take a few tries to find the one that's best for you.

But if you smoke or have other health-risk factors, you're not advised to take the combined Pill past the age of 35. The main risk factors are diabetes, high blood pressure, obesity, migraine, a history of thrombosis or diseases of the heart, gall-bladder or liver. Thrombosis is, fortunately, a rare side effect of the combined Pill; headaches are a lot more common.

If you're in that group, you'll probably be offered a progestogen-only Pill. This is almost as reliable as the combined Pill, as long as you take it at exactly the same time every day. If you take it as little as three hours late, it may not work, and you'll need to use another method, such as condoms, as a back-up until your next bleed. You need to take this into account if you go abroad on holiday, crossing time zones, and it may not suit you if forgetfulness is one of your perimenopausal symptoms.

All forms of hormonal contraception have success rates of 98–99 per cent. This includes pills, implants, injections and the intra-uterine system (IUS), also known as Mirena – a form of intra-uterine device (IUD) containing progestogens. They also make periods lighter, and may stop them altogether. Implants and injections are more likely to cause side effects, including weight gain, headaches, nervousness, acne and depression.

What if you've always preferred more natural forms of contraception and don't want to start taking drugs at this stage, but equally don't want to start again with nappies when your other children are in their teens?

Sterilization is very nearly 100 per cent effective, but is usually irreversible.

The ordinary IUD is 98 per cent successful in preventing pregnancy. It has no side effects, apart from sometimes making periods heavier or more painful, and slightly increasing the risk of infection. An IUD fitted after you're 40 can stay in place till you pass the menopause, and you never have to think about contraception or drug side effects. If one of your perimenopausal symptoms is heavy or painful periods, though, an IUD could make things worse.

Though slightly less guaranteed, barrier methods – caps, diaphragms and male or female condoms – are still more than 90 per cent effective if used correctly.

Natural family planning, using a thermometer or other methods to judge when you're ovulating, can be equally effective. It relies on being very observant and careful, though, and you may find it harder to keep track if the perimenopause makes your periods become irregular. The rhythm method – estimating when your next period is likely to start and then abstaining from sex for a few days around the time of ovulation (14 days before the next period) – is only about 75 per cent effective, and less so if your periods aren't as regular as clockwork.

Not only a woman's problem

Men aren't so constrained by their biological clocks as women are, and can go on fathering children into their nineties. But their sperm quality declines as they get older.

Men's sperm count in industrialized countries has halved during the past 50 years, with pollution as a major suspect. 'Gender-bending' hormone-disrupting chemicals that enter the water supply as industrial waste have been found to produce female characteristics in male fish. Scientists have discovered that other common chemicals also seem to be reducing female fertility.

Sometimes the problem is simple and easily solved. Many men regain their fertility when they stop overheating their sperm by wearing tight trousers, driving a lot, or using a laptop computer. If infertility is a side effect of drugs (legal or illegal) or working in a contaminated environment, a change of lifestyle could sort it out.

Other cases are more difficult. Male infertility can be caused by problems in the testicles, such as a tumour, an infection or a kind of varicose vein called a varicocele. Or it may stem from hormonal or genetic problems. See 'Natural aids to fertility' (below) or, if you're worried, consult your GP.

Are we losing our fertility?

One couple in every six or seven now has difficulty conceiving, according to fertility specialists. Partly this may be because people are starting families later than they did 20 or 30 years ago. Before that time, it's hard to judge how many people had problems conceiving. They rarely sought treatment, as nothing much could be done about it.

But simple biological age isn't the only reason – several factors are involved in the rising incidence of fertility problems:

• Sexually transmitted diseases (STDs), such as chlamydia and gonorrhoea.
• Other health conditions – including digestive disorders such as irritable bowel syndrome (IBS) and coeliac disease.
• Excess weight – two-thirds of Britons are now above a healthy weight. Women on one in-vitro fertilization (IVF) programme were found to be one-third less likely to conceive if they were overweight.
• Being underweight – this reduces fertility even more.
• Damage or growth in the womb and its surroundings, such as ovarian cysts, polycystic ovarian syndrome, fibroids, endometriosis, pelvic inflammatory disease or other infections.
• Genetic factors: paradoxical though it seems, low fertility can be passed from one generation to the next!

Natural aids to fertility

Making simple lifestyle changes can sometimes be just enough to tip the balance in favour of a pregnancy occurring. These changes apply to your partner as well as to you.

• Look at your general working conditions and lifestyle. Do you sleep enough? Miss meals? Spend too much time at a desk? If your fertility is on the borderline, being rundown could reduce your chances of conceiving.
• Give up smoking now, if you haven't already. Smoking reduces fertility in both men and women.
• Don't drink alcohol. A small amount of alcohol in your body at the time of conception may be enough to damage the baby, sometimes in subtle ways that may not show up immediately after birth.
• Reduce your exposure to traffic fumes and chemicals that could have a hormone-disrupting effect (see 'External influences' in Chapter 1 for details).
• Keep your weight within a healthy body-mass index (BMI) range of 20 to 25 (see Chapter 8).
• Eat healthily, with fresh fruit and vegetables as the basis of your diet (see Chapter 8).
• Some nutritionists believe that eating alkaline foods will help if

your cervical mucus is too acidic for sperm to get through. This theory recommends more skimmed milk, bean sprouts and peas, with less red meat and tea, and no Vitamin C supplements.

- Take a 440mg folic acid supplement every day (*he* doesn't have to!). This has been shown to reduce the risk of birth defects such as spina bifida. For both of you, a multivitamin supplement containing the B-complex, C and E may be helpful.

- Try avoiding soya products around the time of ovulation, as there's a possibility that genistein, a component of soya beans, may reduce the likelihood of conception.

- Keep fit, without exercising over-zealously. Over-exercising may reduce your oestrogen levels, prevent ovulation and bring your weight down too far to support a pregnancy. It's just as harmful to his fertility, too.

- Wear loose-fitting clothes and cotton underwear. For him, it keeps sperm at the best temperature for fertility. For you, it reduces your risk of vaginal infections.

- Get him to use a desktop computer, or leave that laptop on the table – if it's on *his* lap, it's heating up his sperm. He should also take showers rather than baths, not too hot, and avoid anything else that could raise the temperature of his sperm. Even driving or riding a bicycle can have an effect.

- See your GP to exclude the possibility of a health condition that is preventing pregnancy, such as bacterial infection in men, endometriosis or fibroids in women (symptoms include menstrual irregularities and abdominal discomfort). You should also check that you (the woman) have rubella immunity – even if you've had a jab, immunity can be lost with time. You may also want genetic counselling if conditions such as cystic fibrosis run in either of your families.

- Try to avoid taking any non-essential drugs. If you take medicine for any condition, consult your GP. Remember that herbal remedies can be as powerful as drugs: some research has suggested that popular supplements such as St John's Wort, echinacea and ginkgo biloba may reduce the ability of sperm to penetrate the egg.

- Consider a course of acupuncture – many couples say it worked for them.

- Having sexual intercourse two or three times a week increases your chance of having sperm ready to fertilize your egg at ovulation.

- Awareness of the fertile times in your cycle can maximize the chances of conception. Consult your GP, family planning clinic, or an organization such as Fertility UK that teaches natural family planning, or the rhythm method.

• It may sound too obvious to state, but check that you're not accidentally doing anything to sabotage your efforts, such as douching, getting overtired or exercising too strenuously.

• Have fun and relax together – stress and tiredness are major obstacles to conception. Surveys show that people work longer hours and have less energy for love-making than ever before. Many people think they're infertile when, in reality, they just haven't given their tired bodies a chance.

'It's quite a scary process'
Kathy, a teacher, went to her doctor after 18 months of trying with her husband for a baby, but didn't get much help and was advised not to worry. 'I think a lot of people find this with their GPs,' she says. 'So we changed GPs.'

The next doctor took them more seriously and, after tests revealed Kathy's hormone levels and her husband's sperm counts were normal, she referred Kathy to a clinic. After a multitude of tests, the specialist found that Kathy's cervical mucus was the wrong pH: it was killing off the sperm.

They were both in their thirties, so despite their concern about high-tech treatments – 'It's quite a scary process, and when you hear about "test-tube babies" you wonder what you're getting into' – they decided to try IVF.

A course of drugs stimulated Kathy's ovaries to produce 23 eggs ('I thought I was going to have a football team'), which were fertilized, frozen and kept for three months to give Kathy's body time to get back to normal. Of the four embryos that were then defrosted, two didn't survive and two were implanted in Kathy's womb but failed to develop. A month later, another four were thawed, but only one survived to be implanted.

After so many disappointments, says Kathy, she hardly dared hope. But this time the pregnancy test was positive, and the couple now have a small daughter. Since then, they've tried to implant some more embryos, but unsuccessfully.

'It would have been nice if our daughter had a brother or sister,' says Kathy, 'but in the end we wanted a child, we've got her and she's wonderful.'

Infertility treatment options

First, your GP can do blood tests to check that you're ovulating, to see if there are any other hormonal problems, and to find out whether you've had rubella. Your partner can have a sperm test and you can both take a urine test for chlamydia. Any of these tests may reveal a simple treatable cause.

If you're referred to a specialist you can have a series of scans, X-rays and keyhole operations to check all your reproductive organs. Your partner will have tests to see how active his sperm is and whether it's able to get through your cervical mucus.

The next stage is assisted conception. Don't be put off by the 'test-tube' image. It's true that it can be gruelling and expensive, as NHS options are limited. The drugs may cause side effects such as heavy periods, nausea, headaches and weight gain. And you face having drug injections, and eggs removed from and replaced in your body under anaesthetic.

But some of the interventions are quite simple. If you're not ovulating, you may be offered hormone tablets or injections that can trigger the release of an egg. If sperm can't get through, you can have intra-uterine insemination (IUI), in which sperm from your partner is put directly into your womb. If the problem is in his sperm, you may be offered sperm from a donor. With all these methods, you can then become pregnant naturally.

The next stage is IVF. You take stronger drugs to produce several eggs at a time; these are then fertilized with sperm from your partner or a donor. Two or more eggs are implanted in your womb, to increase the chances of success, and as a result you have about a 1-in-4 chance of carrying twins or triplets. About 24,000 couples a year have IVF treatment in the UK, and some 8,000 babies are born as a result.

If you are unable to produce suitable eggs even with fertility drugs, you may need to join a waiting list for a donor egg.

If your problem is that the fertilized egg doesn't attach to your womb lining, you may be offered a blastocyst transfer, in which the fertilized egg – now an embryo – is allowed to develop for a few days longer before being placed in your womb, to improve its chance of attaching firmly.

If you've tried IVF unsuccessfully and the problem is in

your partner's sperm, you may be offered intra-cytoplasmic sperm injection (ICSI). It's the same as IVF, except that one egg is taken and injected with one of his sperm before being put in your womb. Like IVF, this has a success rate of 20–30 per cent each time you try.

Costs and problems of infertility treatment

Infertility treatments still have a fairly low success rate and may not be funded by the NHS. Going privately, though, may cost thousands of pounds for each attempt.

Some techniques that help a man with low fertility to become a father may even pass on a tendency to birth defects, as infertile men are ten times more likely than average to carry genetic abnormalities.

Doctors routinely advise people to wait a year or so after giving up contraception before thinking about treatment for infertility. But depending on where you live, you may face a three-year wait for NHS treatment. If you're already in your late thirties, you should start making enquiries within six months – you've nothing to lose by joining a waiting list. Meanwhile, check that you're doing everything you can to improve your chances: see 'Natural aids to fertility' (above).

Keeping a pregnancy safe

Miscarriage is common at any age, but the risk increases sharply after your mid-thirties, and after the age of 40 nearly a quarter of all confirmed pregnancies end in miscarriage, compared with just 1 in 16 before the age of 35.

On the positive side, as an older mother you have several advantages over younger women. You're probably a lot more aware of your body and your health. You may have reached a position at work in which you can negotiate for better conditions, and you're not likely to be involved in dangerous behaviour such as drinking heavily or using illegal drugs.

Almost all the advice in this chapter holds true for supporting a pregnancy as well as beginning one. The only exceptions are any kind of medical treatment (whether orthodox or alternative), such as acupuncture or herbalism. To recap:

- Avoid having any procedure or taking any medicine that's not absolutely necessary. For the same reason, don't take any herbs or food supplements without specialist advice.
- Don't smoke, drink alcohol or take other drugs.
- Avoid infections, another common cause of miscarriage. Avoid contact with anyone who has a cold or other illness. Wash your hands every time you come into the house from outside, as well as before cooking, before eating, after using the loo and after touching houseplants. Don't handle raw meat, cat litter or – if possible – anything dirty.
- Try to keep cool. Anything that makes you too hot can trigger a miscarriage, whether it's sunbathing, taking saunas or running a fever.
- Standing up for a long time can be harmful, as well as overexerting yourself in any way.

Take it easy

Stress is as bad for pregnancy as it is for everything else. Although no one's suggesting a return to the Victorian ideal of resting quietly throughout the pregnancy, women drive themselves too hard in the twenty-first century. Pregnancy isn't a disease, but it is making demands on your body and, for your baby, it's a one-off chance for a strong and healthy start. Putting a lot of energy into other activities could be reducing your baby's share of your resources. Women over 35 are more than twice as likely to suffer a stillbirth, when the baby dies in the womb for no apparent reason, after what seemed like a normal pregnancy. So give yourself time to relax, especially during the final few weeks before the birth.

Finally, if you do miscarry, remember that it shouldn't reduce your chances of success next time. Give yourself time to grieve, and then look forward to the next time. (See *Losing a Baby* by Sarah Ewing, Sheldon Press, 2005.)

5

Baby shock

Many of the women who spoke about their experiences for this book had a first child in their thirties or even forties. They are among the ever-rising number of women who enter the perimenopause at a time when they're adjusting to the demands of motherhood. For some, the collision of these two hormonal forces causes turbulent times.

Women are not only hit with two enormous life changes at once. They're also navigating without maps – few perimenopausal women in previous generations would also have been coping with first babies, jobs and, in some cases, short-term relationships. And, because people live longer, many women find themselves looking after elderly parents as well as small children.

Yet it's a choice more and more women are making: the age at which we're starting families has steadily increased over the past 50 years. In particular, the number of women waiting till they're over 30 to have their first child has risen dramatically.

The under-30 birth rate has been falling for decades, and nearly half of all babies in the UK now are born to women over 30. In much of England, more babies are born to women in their early thirties than in what used to be prime child-bearing time, the early twenties. In Scotland, the over-35 birth rate has doubled since the early 1990s.

Other countries are seeing a similar trend. One Canadian woman in three has her first child in her thirties – a rate that has more than tripled since 1976. In the USA, the number of first-time mothers in their late thirties increased by 36 per cent in the decade to 2001, while the number in their forties rose by 70 per cent. In Sweden, the average age of a first-time mother has soared from little more than 20 to 28 since the 1970s.

The number of women starting a family, or a second family, in their forties is still small, but the early-forties birth rate has doubled since the early 1990s in the UK, accounting for around 1 baby in 50.

'You're more tolerant when you're an older mother'
Annie had her first child at 37 and her second at 40. She sees this as a good time of life to start a family.

'You've established yourself in your job, you're more secure, you've bought the things you need,' she says. 'You've found yourself, so you're quite stable as a person. And because you wanted children so much, you're happy to look after them.'

One symptom she had while the children were small was PMS. 'I used to get very emotional with it,' she says. But it wasn't disastrous. 'You're more mature and tolerant at that age,' she continues. 'You can cope better with things that go wrong.'

Her husband was equally ready to settle down and have children. They share the same attitudes towards child-rearing and the same liberal values, she says, which they've passed on to the children. But that isn't just luck, as they knew each other well enough before starting a family to be certain that they had the same outlook and aspirations.

Neither of them has felt driven to earn a lot of money – Annie works part-time and her husband works for a charity. 'When you're older it's perhaps a less selfish approach,' says Annie. 'You've done most of what you want to do yourself, so you're prepared to put a lot into them.'

All change for midlife motherhood

An older mother is likely to have had many years of freedom, holidays and spending her spare time as she likes. She has probably reached a level at work where she has some control over what she does. She's used to taking responsibility, but in areas that can be negotiated. (Ever tried negotiating with a toddler?) And if a colleague or client threw food in her face, she'd get another job!

We are unimaginably richer and healthier than our relatives of even 60 years ago. But despite our more affluent lifestyles, in many ways new mothers have a tougher time today than in previous generations.

Changing theories of childcare leave them burdened with guilt if they don't create a perfect child-centred environment. And unlike their grandmothers, they don't feel justified in setting rules – something that's extra hard to do if those around you aren't doing it. Mothers today are much less likely than in the past to insist on a set bedtime, for example. One study recently showed that new mothers 30 years ago got an hour and a half more sleep at night than their present-day counterparts. Today's new mums also took twice as long to get their babies settled and were woken up more often during the night.

The 1970s mums also caught up on their sleep by taking a nap when the baby slept during the day, because few of them went out to work. With two incomes being the norm today, even women who want to stay at home for their children's first few years feel the pressure to bring in some cash. And those who do work try to make it up to the children by putting their own needs last on their endless to-do list. An older mother is more likely to set high standards for herself, and castigate herself if she doesn't meet them. Her working-mother guilt makes her reluctant to deny her child anything – especially as this may be the only one she has.

A midlife baby often embodies the realization of a long-held dream. Women who have been in control of their lives for many years often approach pregnancy and childbirth as another project, doing in-depth research and making preparations for the well-planned event. But, as with any dream, the new mother may be devastatingly disappointed by the messy, tiring and sometimes boring reality of childcare. Some of the women who spoke for this book admitted that the reality could never have matched up to their starry-eyed expectations. Having secretly wondered why the mothers around them weren't coping better, they were thrown into shame and depression when their own theories (or books) on childcare let them down. If you're finding things hard, the National Childbirth Trust may be able to help: call 0870 444 8707 to reach volunteers who have gone through difficulties themselves and are happy to talk.

Money often proves more of a problem than expected, especially if you relied on the fact that you would continue to work. Holding down even a part-time job may prove exhausting, and the cost and complications of organizing childcare are a further discouragement. Self-employed women and others who work at home often say they thought they could just get on with their work while the baby was asleep, underestimating the other chores they have to cram into those brief moments, and their sheer tiredness.

For women who loved their work, this can be a difficult time of reassessing priorities. If you'd rather have some time with your baby, work out how much money you could get by on and stick to a tight budget – your baby doesn't care a hoot if he or she lives in secondhand clothes.

Finally, there's the painful truth that some people just don't really enjoy caring for babies. The love just doesn't outweigh the boredom, mess and frustration. This is difficult in any circumstances, but if you've spent years longing for this child, possibly going through arduous medical treatments during your quest, building up a fantasy of the perfect mother-and-baby experience, the disappointment can be shattering.

Pregnancy itself may be more complicated than you'd envisaged. Problems such as high blood pressure or bleeding in the third trimester are nearly twice as likely after 35 as before 30. Also, studies have found that doctors are more likely to intervene in a birth if the mother is over 35, even if she's not in any trouble, just because they're worried about her age. So she's more likely to have an induced labour, a forceps delivery or even a Caesarean. For help around the period of birth and afterwards, contact the National Childbirth Trust (see Useful addresses at the back of this book).

And, while older mothers are more likely to breastfeed, giving their baby the best start in life, it's easy to be derailed by wrong advice; also, perimenopausal breast tenderness and nipple soreness can make this difficult. Talk to your health visitor or contact the Breastfeeding Network and La Leche League (see Useful addresses). Look for a Baby Café near you (see Useful addresses) for a tea break with breastfeeding advice in friendly company with other breastfeeding mums.

'You think when you've had three, the experience should help you cope'
Sheila was the mother of three teenage boys when she had her fourth son at the age of 36.

'It was like starting again with the last one,' she says. 'It seemed harder than bringing up the other three together, perhaps because of the age difference.'

She and her husband tried to treat them all fairly, but, says Sheila, 'Perhaps we spoilt him more because he was the last one. He had more attention, even though we tried to give the same to each of them.'

A keen runner when she was younger, Sheila found she had no time for exercise after her last son was born.

'I got more stressed with the last one,' she says. 'You think when you've had three, the experience should help you cope. I did cope, but it was more stressful. Now it's nice to have the grandchildren for a while and then pass them back!'

Baby shock tactics

Make life a little easier for yourself, with some tips from women who've been there too:

- Accept all offers of help, and ask for more if you're not getting enough.

- Let go of any 'perfect mother, perfect baby' fantasies.
- Learn from your baby to live in the moment. You'll both gain more if you enjoy what you're doing right now, even if it's not what you'd planned, rather than struggling to achieve something that's out of reach.
- If you're feeling stressed or unhappy, talk to your husband/ partner, friends and family. (Use the information in Chapter 3.) But if it continues for more than a few days, or if you feel desperate, seek help from your GP or health visitor. Don't let depression become a habit – it will harm your baby and yourself.
- Coping with any perimenopausal symptoms can give you more energy to put into motherhood. Use the advice in this book, and go to your GP or well-woman clinic if necessary.
- Spend time with other mothers like yourself. If you feel out of place with mums in their twenties, look or advertise for a local group of older mothers.
- Online groups, books and forums can be a lifeline. (See Useful addresses and Further reading – in particular, the book *Hot Flashes, Warm Bottles: First-Time Mothers over Forty* by Nancy London.)

Am I flushing, or has my toddler set fire to the curtains?

With all that has been written about women starting a family in their thirties or later, not much has been said about the challenges raised by this period of life overlapping with the run-up to the menopause.

It comes as a shock to suffer a hot flush while you're trying to tempt a toddler away from the sweet shelf. And any woman who is offered hormone replacement therapy (HRT) when she's still hoping to have another child will want to know a lot more before making a decision.

One thing almost every mother of this age reports is the exhaustion – a level of tiredness that they had never previously imagined. Parents of small children often have to survive on less sleep than they thought possible, which can leave a fit 25-year-old feeling wrecked. But as you approach 40, it becomes harder to function without adequate rest. (See Chapter 7 for tips on sleep.)

Tiredness is part of the perimenopause for many women, even without new demands on their energy. Sharing your bed with the baby is cosy and convenient for feeding, though you need to weigh this against an increased risk of infant death, especially if you smoke or drink. But if you're kicked awake ten times a night, please give yourself a break and put the baby in a cot beside you. A baby also generates heat like a little radiator, increasing your risk of night sweats disturbing your sleep.

The heavy bleeding that so many women experience early in the perimenopause just adds to the exhaustion. At least that's one factor that can be cured: get your GP to check if you're anaemic, and see Chapters 6 and 8 for advice on countering heavy bleeding.

In addition, many older mothers admit that their sex lives are now a dim memory, and can hardly imagine their libido ever returning. This often happens during the perimenopause, but it is exacerbated by tiredness and the demands of childcare. This can affect women at any age after a birth, especially if it was difficult. The information in Chapter 3 may help, but nothing is more valuable than a loving partner, so don't let the intimacy and communication die away – this phase doesn't last for ever.

One of the most disorientating features of midlife motherhood is having a hot flush – the visible symbol of menopause in most people's eyes – while cradling a baby. It can give rise to powerful emotions. Suddenly you feel like an intruder in babyland, wondering if you seem ridiculous, questioning whether you've taken on something you should have left alone. As stress can trigger a hot flush, it's not surprising that this may happen when you're trying to soothe a crying baby or calm an enraged toddler. Trying to get things done in a hurry can set one off too. Heat is of course a factor – even holding a clingy child or overheating the house (harmful for a baby too) can bring on a hot flush.

The mood swings and PMS symptoms of early perimenopause, combined with the demands of new motherhood, can be mistaken for postnatal depression. Do push yourself to try healthy eating and aerobic exercise, but if symptoms persist consult your GP.

As an older mother, you're more likely to suffer from back pain, exacerbated by carrying a baby and all its accoutrements. You can reduce the risk of damage by squatting rather than leaning down to pick up the baby, thus letting your legs rather than your back take the strain. (See Chapter 7 for more ways to take care of your back.)

Heavy legs and aching joints, which affect many women during the perimenopause, make it hard to play with a lively child. Try to sit down as much as possible rather than standing. If you're comfortable lying on the floor, children enjoy games that you can join in at their level. And don't be too puritanical about children's television and

DVDs: watching them together is an activity you can share while taking a mental and physical break.

Hormones can scramble your brain: mental fuzziness strikes many women during pregnancy, and it's one of the most unnerving symptoms of perimenopause too. Don't blame yourself if you take your baby's toy bag to work and leave your work bag with the childminder. Just try to organize things to make life easier. Allow yourself more time to get ready, if possible, and help yourself with visual cues such as notes on the fridge. But don't do anything that you just don't feel up to: driving is dangerous if your mind isn't totally on the road.

Perimenopausal clumsiness is frightening when you're in charge of a small child. Many women report being afraid they would trip and drop the baby, or fall on top of her. Being stressed or in a hurry makes these things worse, so remember some of your advantages: you're older and wiser, you know that taking things slowly achieves them faster, and basically if you break a few plates it's not the end of the world.

'I sometimes feel selfish for having had her so late'
Helen could hardly have been in better shape when she had her daughter Katie, at the age of 44, after eight years of trying. Eating wholefoods, taking long walks, practising yoga and cycling everywhere, she had lived a holistic lifestyle for decades and was probably fitter than most women in their thirties. But the perimenopause hit hard when she was at home with a baby.

'I hardly used to notice periods before,' she says. 'Now I get a two-day headache that really wipes me out, and nothing seems to touch it. I have persistent mouth ulcers too.'

A recent fall left her with joints that wouldn't stop aching, making it an ordeal to pick up her little daughter. But symptoms that would annoy anyone, such as occasional bouts of dizziness, are more frightening when you're responsible for a small child. She now feels less confident of her balance, especially riding her bike with her daughter on the back.

'I'm so sensitive to everything,' adds Helen. 'I can't deal with stress, which is difficult when you've got a child who wants 100 per cent attention. The brain goes as well – I'll be telling her a story, something interrupts me and I won't have a clue what I was saying.'

Her healthy lifestyle went down the drain: she and her husband grab a ready meal from the freezer instead of cooking when they've got Katie to bed. Helen now takes supplements to replace some of the nutrients she's missing.

Helen enjoys the kinship she feels with mothers whom she wouldn't have met otherwise. Her age doesn't make as much difference as she expected, as so many women now start families in their thirties. But she sympathizes with her neighbour, who had her second child at 45, and went through even more exhaustion with a teenager and a toddler.

'The ten years between 35 and 45 make an enormous difference,' says Helen. 'I really wish I'd done it earlier.'

It's the tiredness that makes the biggest impact on her life. 'I'm tired all the time. All I crave is some time to myself and enough sleep. When you're younger you can manage with little sleep, but I need recovery time now, and I can't get it. I feel I ought to have more time for her, and I'm always feeling guilty that I'm not doing it properly.

'It's great if you can join in at her level, and I sometimes can. But you have to have the energy to put into being in her lovely fantasy world, talking about unicorns and princesses.

'I sometimes feel selfish for having had her so late. But in spite of all my moans and groans, I'm glad I've got her. You can't imagine the love you feel, that overwhelms anything else. I wouldn't change it.'

'I wouldn't have done it differently'

This is a common saying among older mothers, for starting a family after 35 has much to be said for it. You've fulfilled a lot of your youthful ambitions and let go of some of the others. You're no longer desperate to take part in every new sensation, and you've probably grown out of the restlessness and hedonism that quite naturally ruled your earlier life.

You're not only more financially secure, but more emotionally stable too. With luck, you've mellowed to the stage where you can smile at the sort of setbacks – a nappy disaster as you leave the house, baby food rubbed into your CD collection – that would have driven you mad 20 years ago. If you're happily settled in a relationship and both of you are ready for parenthood, this is a wonderful time.

Older mothers are usually more patient, and have the experience to know that small accidents and setbacks don't matter as long as no one is injured. Statistics show that they're likely to be more educated and affluent than younger mothers. They're often delighted to take a break from employment to spend time in a new and more creative endeavour. And instead of resenting their lost freedom, they're likely to welcome the new sense of groundedness.

Even history is on their side. Despite all the press concern about the dangers of late motherhood, women today aren't doing anything unprecedented. It's true that we're settling down later than our parents did – but they were the ones who bucked the trend by marrying and having children early. Up till the 1940s, women were starting families at about the same age, on average, as they do now. Then came the postwar baby boom, when family life was top of everyone's agenda and people started marrying and having children at an earlier age.

Even having children over the age of 40 isn't unusual, although only 6,000 women over 40 had babies in 1977. In 1964, when the birth rate peaked, 23,000 babies were born to women over 40, compared with 15,000 in 2000.

It's true that most midlife mothers in the past weren't also coping with jobs and caring for elderly parents (who would probably have died earlier). On the other hand, they didn't have any labour-saving devices – laundry alone could take an entire day of heavy work.

And historical research shows that women who had children in their forties went on to live longer than the average, possibly because it was a sign that their biological clock was ticking slowly.

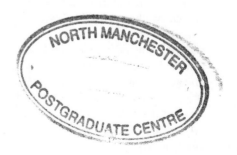

6

HRT and other medical help

As the perimenopause isn't a disease, most women don't need medicine. But like any other transition, it can cause upheaval. As certain drugs may help with some symptoms, it's worth knowing what's available.

The treatment we all think of in relation to this time of life is hormone replacement therapy (HRT). It has also been widely used by women who have passed the menopause, seeking to fend off the ills of old age such as osteoporosis and heart disease. And it is increasingly being offered to younger women in early perimenopause.

HRT offers proven benefits for some symptoms, mainly those that arise near the end of the perimenopause. But it doesn't suit everyone, and there are safety questions over its use before and after that time.

Recent studies have even shown it to cause more harm than good in certain areas. Yet some women swear by it. Causing even more confusion, the latest research seems to change the picture week by week.

So why is there so much disagreement about the benefits and risks of HRT?

The HRT story

In a 1963 paper entitled 'The Fate of the Nontreated Post-Menopausal Woman: A Plea for the Maintenance of Adequate Estrogen from Puberty to the Grave', New York gynaecologist Dr Robert A. Wilson painted a heart-rending portrait of 'the untold misery of alcoholism, drug addiction, divorce and broken homes caused by these unstable, estrogen-starved women'.

Ladies who had seen middle age as a time to loosen their corsets and play golf may have wondered what they'd been missing out on. But the doctors were serious: menopause was not only unhealthy but unnatural – and they were going to conquer it.

For a long time, all women's midlife changes continued to be bundled under the heading of 'the menopause'. If any treatment was offered, it was one-size-fits-all: HRT. Originally this was oestrogen alone, as the symptoms of the perimenopause were all thought to be caused by declining levels of this one hormone. Doctors didn't realize that this increased the risk of uterine cancer until, sadly, numerous women had died as a result.

The next formulations contained progestogens (also known as progestins), synthetic copies of the hormone progesterone. This was meant to reduce the health risks from oestrogen while still easing the symptoms. Because some of the symptoms were actually caused by loss of progesterone, this did help some women. But many others found that the progestogens themselves caused unwelcome side effects.

There was a colossal drop-out rate as women struggled with side effects and tried to find a formulation that helped more than it hindered. Yet some women seemed to thrive on HRT, and continued taking it for years. So the ones who didn't thrive thought they just hadn't found the right drug or dosage.

Looking at our physiology makes it easier to understand what was going on. Our bodies are constantly at work producing tiny quantities of hormones and other chemicals, endlessly carrying out adjustments at an infinitesimal scale, making changes on the basis of what we're doing, what we're eating, what's happening around us, even what's going through our minds.

Attempting to replicate this with a drug is an almost ludicrously difficult task. Drugs work like a blunt instrument compared with the laser precision of the body's natural processes.

When the natural processes go wrong, and we become ill, that blunt instrument may be all we have to help us. Some drugs, such as antibiotics, are life-savers: they have a simple task to do, in killing an invading organism, and they do it magnificently. But when drugs attempt to tackle a more complicated problem, their task is a lot more difficult and correspondingly less often successful.

Researchers are understandably excited at finding a drug that will, apparently, replace an element in the body that's no longer working as it used to. But in their enthusiasm they overlook the other elements that worked in conjunction with it, and the processes that won't necessarily work so well with the replacement.

Oestrogen, for example, helps protect young women from heart disease – but the latest research suggests that when taken after menopause it has the opposite effect, because its good effects only happen in conjunction with two other chemicals which also decline during the perimenopause.

Added to this is the amount of time it takes to find out what effect a drug is having. It took years for an increasing rate of uterine cancer to be first measured, then linked with oestrogen replacement. Over the decades, HRT has been hailed as the solution to all kinds of problems, from perimenopausal symptoms to the ills of old age. One by one these claims have fallen, as HRT proved either ineffective or actually harmful.

Late in 2004, the Royal College of Obstetricians and Gynaecologists issued new advice that women should only take HRT for short-term relief of severe symptoms, and that the risks of taking it in the long term outweighed the benefits.

'I couldn't cope with the flooding'
Patricia didn't think twice before taking HRT. She'd been on the Pill since her twenties, swapping to the progestogen-only version in her mid-thirties, without any problems. So when she started getting hot flushes, she was well disposed towards what seemed like another hormonal helper.

As soon as she began taking HRT, she started having heavy periods, for the first time in her life. She put up with it at first, but when she started flooding at work, she went back to her GP.

'I asked my GP for a different prescription but he refused to change it,' says Patricia.

She was determined to persevere, but the heavy periods got longer until she was bleeding for up to two weeks a month. Feeling tired and lethargic all the time, she went back to her GP again. This time he prescribed antidepressants. She took these too, though they made her throat feel parched.

'One day I had some foreign students coming to stay and I had to collect them at 6 a.m.,' she says. 'I knew I couldn't cope with the flooding so I stopped taking the HRT a few days before.' It was nearly two years since she had started taking HRT. 'I stopped the antidepressants too,' she says, 'and I started feeling better almost at once.'

Since then, she says, she feels much more energetic, backing her view that the symptoms were at least partly caused by heavy blood loss.

Patricia gave up her endless efforts to organize the chaotic office where she earned her living, and found she could live on part-time work. Instead of struggling through more hours at the office, she now augments her wages by selling short stories and is completing a novel.

'Often the perimenopause strikes at a time when women are going through changes at home and at work, and they find themselves worrying about symptoms they wouldn't give a damn about if things were going smoothly,' she says. She still has hot flushes, but they don't bother her – in fact, she calls them 'power surges' and says they can be invigorating.

'They clear my head like a sniff of smelling salts,' she says. 'If a worrying thought comes into my mind I get an instant power surge and then I feel better. If I'm feeling a bit muzzy I do it deliberately.

'For a while I was waking up in the night with everything aching, but that's eased off since I went back to taking exercise every day.'

Worrying new evidence about HRT

Although drugs have to go through a number of trials before they are allowed on to the market, the tests can be carried out or sponsored by the manufacturers, who are not obliged to reveal any unfavourable results.

Universities and government organizations can carry out tests of their own – and this is where most of the evidence against a drug is likely to come out. But research into finding and testing new drugs is very expensive. That's why it's mainly carried out by drug companies, which then need to recoup the money they've spent with big sales.

The amount of government money spent on independent research has fallen steeply since the 1970s, meaning that even research carried out at universities is often paid for by drug companies. Although the big charities also spend a lot on independent research, it's only into the areas that they cover – cancer, heart disease and a few of the other major conditions. That leaves many other possible effects not being investigated.

Consequently, drugs have often been in use for some time before harmful effects start showing up. At that stage, governments may step in and do some independent research.

In 2003, the UK's Million Women study, which had followed more than a million women aged 50-plus for over a decade, reported that use of HRT had led to 20,000 extra deaths from breast cancer. Combined HRT seemed to be more of a risk for breast cancer than oestrogen alone. Later the same year, a Swedish study was stopped early, after finding that women who had survived breast cancer were nearly four times more likely to develop another breast tumour if they used HRT. This was bad news. Although people had suspected there might be a link between HRT and breast cancer, this had never been supported by drug-company evidence.

More of a shock came from studies, both by drug companies and by health organizations, into claims that HRT improved women's health after the menopause. In 1998 the US Heart and Estrogen/ Progestin Replacement Study (HERS) of post-menopausal women with heart disease found, unexpectedly, that combined HRT seemed to increase their health risks rather than reducing them.

In 2002 the follow-up study to this, HERS-2, confirmed that the women with heart disease who took combined HRT were more likely to suffer a blood clot or gall-bladder disease than those who took a placebo, or dummy pill. And although HRT improved their cholesterol levels, it didn't reduce their risk of having a heart attack.

What about women without existing heart disease? Another massive US study called the Women's Health Initiative (WHI) had recruited 27,000 healthy post-menopausal women in 1991. It aimed to find out the effects of taking either oestrogen alone, or combined HRT, or a placebo.

In 2004 the WHI study was stopped, earlier than planned, after researchers realized that the dangers of taking HRT so far outweighed any benefits that they could not justify the risks to their volunteers. Oestrogen alone was found to give no protection against heart disease, and it increased the risk of a stroke.

The branch of the WHI study using combined HRT, which had been stopped in 2002, found that women were less likely than before to suffer colon cancer or a broken bone (bones become weaker as oestrogen levels fall). But their risk of suffering heart disease, strokes, blood clots, dementia and breast cancer had increased.

Another US study, the Women's Estrogen for Stroke Trial, found that oestrogen didn't benefit older women who had had a stroke. In fact, if they had another stroke, it was likely to be worse if they had taken oestrogen. Early in 2005, researchers at the University of Nottingham reviewed studies involving 40,000 women and found their risk of suffering a stroke, if they took HRT, increased by 29 per cent.

One study even found that older women on HRT had poorer hearing than those not on it, although researchers had thought (because the ear contains oestrogen receptors) that HRT should have a positive effect on hearing.

Weighing up the risks and benefits of HRT for yourself

The following question has been asked: did the drug companies not know the potential risks of HRT when they put the drugs on the market?

Independent research by doctors at Oxford University and a Finnish national health institute had published a study in 1997 claiming that women on HRT had a higher risk of heart disease. This went so much against the grain of current belief that their research was widely rejected – until the WHI study confirmed their results. The doctors went through the courts to gain access to drug-company research, and revealed, in the *British Medical Journal* in 2004, that some drug companies too had known, or suspected, the risks for many years.

Doctors try to use what they call 'evidence-based medicine', meaning treatments that have been proved safe and effective. But with new drugs, this information is based on published drug trials, which we now know may tell only part of the story. The system means that it's hard to know what's safe and effective until it's been used by a large number of human patients.

We may resent being used as guinea pigs, but until governments pay for independent research we have to rely on what drug companies let us know. As that's not about to happen, what should we do in the meantime?

Most of the evidence about HRT's risks come from studies of older women. They were using HRT after the menopause, either because they were still getting hot flushes (which often continue for a few years afterwards) or to try to prevent the ills of old age. All the evidence shows that HRT isn't a good course for them, unless the menopausal symptoms are so unbearable that they'd rather take the risk.

There's not a lot of independent information about the effects on younger women of taking it during the few years of the perimenopause. From what we know at present, though, it seems likely that taking HRT for just three or four years should not greatly increase the risk of serious diseases, as long as you're healthy and have no family history of them.

The breast-cancer risk seems to be temporary, in that five years after you stop taking HRT you have no more risk than you had before you started it. But it's still probably safest not to use HRT if you, or a close relative, have had cancer of the breast, endometrium (womb lining) or uterus, or if you have liver disease, or if you have ever had a blood clot – for example, when you were pregnant or on the Pill.

Advice from the UK government's Committee on Safety of Medicines is to use the lowest effective dose for as short a time as possible. A major medical conference on the subject recently gave the same advice, and concluded that the best person to take HRT was a young, healthy woman suffering from severe perimenopausal symptoms. It's no longer recommended as a long-term anti-ageing therapy, or as an effort to prevent any of the diseases of old age.

Where HRT can help

The disadvantages of HRT don't rule it out as a treatment. Although the risks are genuine, they're not enormous if you're otherwise healthy and have no family history of the diseases HRT promotes. And it can be very helpful for women who are badly affected, especially by the vasomotor symptoms: hot flushes and night sweats. It can also solve the problems of heavy bleeding, urinary infections and vaginal dryness, and reduce depression.

If you're having hot flushes several times a day, you may not care about the long-term effects of anything that gives you your life back now. The risk of death from HRT is relatively small – far less than from smoking, for example. And if you're living through hormone hell, you may well feel it's worth the risk. Only you can make that decision.

If your GP or well-woman clinic are reasonable, they'll be happy for you to experiment to find the lowest possible dose that keeps your symptoms under control.

It's not the fear of illness in the future that puts many women off using HRT. Most of those who try it give up after a few months because of the side effects. These include vaginal discharge, bleeding at odd times, headaches, nausea, swollen breasts and fluid retention. But there are numerous different formulations available, using different forms of oestrogen or of progestogen, and different strengths. If your perimenopausal symptoms are severe, it's worth trying several brands of HRT to find one that does the job without side effects.

HRT can be used in various different forms: as tablets, skin patches, skin gel, pellets implanted under your skin, or even a nasal spray called Aerodiol. You need a higher dose of oestrogen with tablets than with the other products, as tablets have to go through your digestive system before reaching their mark. Some women find the other products irritate their skin; it's a question of finding a method that suits you.

Oestrogen-only brands – such as Premarin, Estraderm and Evorel – tend to control the symptoms more effectively and cause fewer side effects than those combined with progestogens. If your main problem is vaginal dryness, leading to soreness and painful sex, you can use a vaginal tablet, ring or cream. Very little will go as far as your bloodstream, so it won't have much effect on other symptoms. But oestrogen is not usually prescribed alone, except to women who have had a hysterectomy, because of the increased risk of cancer. Even if you're just using a vaginal product, you're advised to take a progestogen tablet.

Most prescriptions are for combined HRT – such as Nuvelle, Premique and Prempak-C. While you're still having periods, you're most likely to be offered cyclical HRT, in which you have oestrogen every day with a progestogen added during the final 10 to 14 days of the 28-day cycle. You'll probably get a monthly bleed similar to a fairly light period.

Continuous HRT, containing both oestrogen and progestogen every day, prevents bleeding but is usually only offered to women who have already gone through the menopause.

The hormones in HRT are not always identical to those in your body. They may contain conjugated oestrogen made from pregnant mares' urine, or estrified oestrogen from plants, or synthetic oestrogen made in a laboratory. The progestogens are mainly synthetic, although there's a school of thought that considers these to be unhelpful as they're too unlike the body's own hormone, progesterone.

Early in the perimenopause

HRT can be helpful, especially for hot flushes and night sweats. Some women get these early in the perimenopause. But they're most common towards the end, for the few years before and after periods stop, when oestrogen levels are low and falling.

It's important to remember that, in the early stages of the perimenopause, symptoms are probably not caused by simple lack of oestrogen. They may be caused by fluctuating oestrogen levels, which can even be high, along with low progesterone levels. This is probably the case if you're having PMS-like symptoms and frequent heavy periods, your vaginal mucus is stretchy, and your breasts are swollen or lumpy.

The progestogen component of HRT may not be similar enough to your own progesterone to help, and you don't need extra oestrogen if you're already producing plenty – indeed, it could be harmful.

'Natural progesterone' (manufactured from a plant, but identical to the human hormone) is claimed by some doctors to help more, during the early perimenopause, than HRT. It is not widely used, as the body breaks it down faster than progestogens, but your doctor may prescribe vaginal progesterone gels called Crinone or Cyclogest. A 20mg progesterone cream spread on the skin has been shown to reduce troublesome vasomotor symptoms, hot flushes and night sweats, in one study in which women used a quarter of a teaspoonful.

Natural progesterone or progestogens have long been prescribed to treat PMS, although one study published in the *British Medical Journal* in 2001 found that it worked no better than a placebo.

Other medicines

HRT isn't the only drug that can help relieve perimenopausal symptoms, especially the vasomotor symptoms of hot flushes and night sweats, so you may wish to try other medicines first.

The 'male' hormone, testosterone, is claimed by some researchers to relieve hot flushes and increase women's sex drive. Women do naturally produce small amounts of testosterone, and levels of this decrease during the perimenopause. There's little evidence that taking testosterone works as claimed, but you may think it's worth a try. It can be delivered as an implant under your skin, as capsules (Restandol), a skin patch (Andropatch) and in the form of injections.

A drug called clonidine, usually prescribed to treat high blood pressure or migraine, may help reduce hot flushes, though there isn't yet much evidence about its effects in this area. It is prescribed in tablet form under the names Catapres or Dixarit. Side effects may include drowsiness, dizziness, constipation or a dry mouth.

Tibolone (Livial), a hormone-like drug, has been found to relieve hot flushes and vaginal dryness, as well as restoring sex drive. But because it causes bleeding if you still have periods, it is usually only prescribed for women past the menopause. It was discovered in 2005 to cause a slightly increased risk of endometrial cancer.

Selective serotonin-reuptake inhibitors (SSRIs) may reduce depression and hot flushes, in low doses, but can cause mood swings and reduce your sex drive, and have been linked with dangerous side effects including suicidal impulses (see Chapter 3).

Some doctors recommend taking a low-dose combined Pill, even if you don't need it for contraceptive purposes. It can relieve heavy bleeding and reduce the number and severity of hot flushes. Many women find that it helps with other perimenopausal symptoms too (see Chapter 4 for more details).

HRT in a nutshell

- Combined HRT can help with troublesome symptoms such as hot flushes.
- Take the lowest dose that helps, and for as short a time as possible.
- It increases the short-term risk of some problems, such as deep-vein thrombosis.
- Oestrogen alone may have fewer side effects, but increases the risk of uterine and possibly endometrial cancer. It is not prescribed unless you have had a hysterectomy.
- In the long term, HRT is unlikely to prevent any disease and has been found to increase the risk of some serious conditions.

7

Complementary remedies and self-help

The perimenopausal transition can be a bumpy ride at times, but can be smoothed out with lifestyle management and self-help techniques. For some people, natural remedies often prove gentler and more effective than drugs.

The two most proven forms of self-help for perimenopausal symptoms are healthy eating and exercise (see Chapters 8 and 9). But if your hormones are fluctuating severely, healthy eating and exercise may not be enough, especially if you suffer that perimenopausal bugbear: hot flushes. Although more often expected towards the end of the perimenopause, many women encounter them at the beginning. Urinary incontinence is another unwelcome symptom that is not really affected by diet and exercise. Luckily, it responds to other self-help measures.

The remedies in this chapter can all be used in conjunction with a healthy eating and exercise programme, but some herbal remedies interact with drugs, so check with your doctor if you're taking any other medicines (see box entitled 'Safety first').

When you're using complementary or alternative medicine (CAM), try to use the treatment regularly as you would if taking a medicinal drug. If your symptoms haven't responded within a reasonable time (up to three months for herbs and food supplements), try a different remedy. But don't be a martyr to the cause of complementary therapies: if these don't work for you and your symptoms are a nuisance, do visit your GP. The days are long past when women felt they had to suffer in silence.

(*Note*: If you have severe pain or any other symptom that worries you, don't use CAM remedies but go straight to your GP. The same applies if you develop heavy or prolonged bleeding, or periods less than three weeks apart, or renewed bleeding after more than a year without periods.)

Evidence concerning CAM

Until the 1990s, it was hard to say whether CAM remedies worked or not. Many people found them useful, but there was very little published evidence to show whether they worked in themselves or simply had a placebo effect. Unlike drugs, which have to be found both effective and harmless before they can be legally prescribed, CAM remedies could be sold with no backing evidence at all, although manufacturers weren't allowed to make health claims on the labels. Drug-type trials are enormously expensive, and most of the smaller manufacturers of CAM remedies and food supplements simply couldn't afford to do them.

Safety first

If a remedy is strong enough to affect physical symptoms, it is strong enough to cause possible side effects. Of all branches of CAM, herbalism – one of the most effective – is the most dangerous. Every year, herbal remedies cause more adverse effects than all other branches of CAM put together, and these sometimes lead to liver failure and death.

Be very wary of home-made remedies unless you're sure the person making them knows what they're doing; paper qualifications don't always mean a lot. If you're taking a proprietary brand, use something from a major pharmacy or other well-established firm. Take no more than the recommended dosage. Check with your doctor that it's safe if you're taking any other medicines, and don't use herbal remedies if you may be pregnant, unless they're specifically made for use in pregnancy.

Don't use remedies that could have oestrogenic effects – such as black cohosh, red clover or phytoestrogen tablets – if you're taking HRT.

As the market for CAM remedies took off during the 1980s and 1990s, CAM companies started putting money into providing evidence for their goods. Consequently, there is now quite a lot of published evidence for some of them. At the same time, much evidence for new drugs has been brought into doubt, as pharmaceutical companies have been found to have suppressed the results of trials that showed their products either didn't work or were harmful.

Drugs are still far more regulated than the CAM market, and have to contain exactly what the makers claim. Consumer studies analysing CAM remedies, though, often turn up products that contain less than the amount stated on the label, or an inferior version of the active ingredient – or occasionally even something totally different. Results of these analyses are hard to get hold of. The consumers' magazine *Which?* sometimes produces a report on the subject, and a magazine called *Proof!* regularly tests several different brands of the same remedy.

If you try a remedy and it doesn't work for you, it's worth trying to find out if there's a better brand available. In general (though this isn't infallible), you get what you pay for, and well-known companies have a reputation to keep up. When studies are published showing the effectiveness of a particular remedy, such as evening primrose oil or ginkgo biloba, try to find out what formulation or dosage was used, and whether it was a named brand. Every other company producing the same remedy will jump on the bandwagon, but you can only be sure that the evidence applies to the brand or formulation used in the trial.

The phytoestrogen story

Phytoestrogens are CAM's best-known answer to perimenopausal symptoms. They are the plant version of oestrogen, and have some of that hormone's effects on the body – mostly beneficial, according to the research so far. They come in several forms. Isoflavones, the best known and most studied, are abundant in soya beans and other legumes such as lentils and chickpeas. Lignans are found in linseed (flaxseed), sunflower seeds, wholegrain cereals and some fruit and vegetables, including apples and onions. Sprouted soya beans and alfalfa are sources of coumestans.

Phytoestrogens are most effective against hot flushes and night sweats, though there's some evidence that they may also help against insomnia, headaches and nervousness.

Soya is the most popular source of phytoestrogens for women seeking relief from hot flushes. French researchers, for example, found that two-thirds of women taking a 70mg soya isoflavone preparation called Phyto Soya found they were having only half as many hot flushes by the end of the four-month trial. Several other studies have found similar effects.

But there has been some concern about the way this oriental staple is used in the West. The Chinese and Japanese traditionally eat soya in the form of beancurd (tofu) and fermented pastes such as miso. In the West we've taken it up with gusto, not only swallowing it in capsule form as a supplement, but also producing all kinds of new soya-based food products. Some researchers are concerned that we don't know enough about the results of eating soya in this way, partly because it means we're taking it in concentrated forms and larger amounts than in the well-studied traditional diet. One concern is that it could affect the thyroid, which can also be affected by the hormonal changes of the perimenopause.

On the other hand, many women with troublesome vasomotor symptoms have found soya foods helpful. The answer may be to eat soya foods, as far as possible, as Chinese and Japanese women do, cooking with beancurd and soya pastes.

Although phytoestrogens haven't been proved to increase the risk of hormone-dependent cancers, there's still a lot of research to be done. It would be wise not to have more than one or two servings a day if you've had one of these cancers or are in a high-risk group.

'I had to give it time to work'

Maria was in her late thirties and had never heard of the perimenopause when she went to her GP with a painful lump in her breast.

'I was terrified,' she says. 'I thought it was cancer – I suppose that's the first thing you think of. The GP said it was probably harmless, as she could feel some lumpiness in both breasts, but, as she said afterwards, that's no guarantee.'

After a mammogram and a biopsy showed that there was no sign of cancer, Maria was surprised that her doctor prescribed evening primrose oil to relieve the pain.

'I'd heard of it, but only as an alternative remedy,' she says. 'I didn't realize you could get it on the NHS. I took it for a few weeks and it didn't help, so I got out of the habit of taking it every day and eventually stopped altogether. Next time I saw the GP, more than a year later, she asked about it and I said I'd given up, but still had the breast pain. She advised me to try again, but this time give it three months to work. I did, and it started working in less than that time. I hadn't given it enough of a chance before.'

When evening primrose oil stopped being available on the NHS, Maria simply started buying it from a health-food shop.

'I haven't had any other symptoms,' she says. 'I don't know whether that's because of the evening primrose oil or not. But it's really good for my skin too, so I'd keep it up for that if nothing else!'

Alternative hormone regulators – what's the evidence?

Black cohosh (Actaea racemosa or Cimicifuga racemosa)
Several studies have revealed the effectiveness of this powerful herb in countering perimenopausal symptoms, especially hot flushes and sweating. Most of the studies have used a German preparation called Remifemin, at doses of 40–80mg a day (two to four tablets). In some cases it proved as effective as HRT, and in most it was better than a placebo.

The studies followed women using black cohosh for up to six months, but there is no information about using it in the longer term. Don't use it if you have high blood pressure or are sensitive to aspirin, and make sure you're not pregnant before taking this herb, as it can harm babies in the womb. There has also been one case of a woman suffering liver failure after taking a black cohosh remedy; and as with any strong herb, don't take it in conjunction with medicines that could also put a strain on your liver: check with your GP if you are taking anything else. Otherwise, only a few minor side effects have been reported, usually headaches, heaviness in the legs or stomach upsets.

It's not yet clear whether the herb has oestrogenic effects or works in some other way. Although it is not thought to promote the growth of cancers, there is no proof of this, so you're advised not to take black cohosh if you have had breast cancer or any other condition that can be exacerbated by oestrogen.

Dong quai (Angelica sinensis)
This popular Chinese herb, believed to regulate hormones and stimulate libido, is traditionally used as part of a prescription tailor-made for an individual after a consultation with a herbalist. This one ingredient would not normally be taken alone. The prescription may vary according to numerous factors, including your constitution and the weather as well as your precise symptoms.

Studies carried out on dong quai alone have had mixed results, but some have found that it may relieve hot flushes. It is believed to increase the menstrual flow, so should not be taken during a period. It may increase sensitivity to sun and (for good and bad) reduce the blood's ability to clot.

Red clover (Trifolium pratense)
This source of isoflavones has been claimed to reduce the incidence of hot flushes, though there is not yet a lot of evidence to back this.

The recommended dose is 40mg, and a product called Promensil, containing this amount, has been used in several studies.

Chasteberry (Vitex agnus castus)

This herbal remedy has been proved to alleviate breast pain and the PMS-like symptoms of perimenopause at a dose of 20mg a day. Because it has progesterone-like effects, it should not be used with any hormonal drug, such as HRT or the cancer medicine tamoxifen, and it may reduce the effectiveness of the contraceptive Pill. Few adverse effects have been reported, but they may include stomach upsets, rashes and bleeding between periods.

Evening primrose oil

Many women find this useful throughout their reproductive life, especially to counter breast pain and PMS. Studies have also shown that it relieves skin conditions such as eczema, which suggests that it might help with perimenopausal itchiness. It contains plenty of the fatty acid GLA, and is said to help the body use both that and other nutrients, such as calcium, more effectively. Two of the most studied brands are Efamol and Epogam. If you suffer from epilepsy or manic-depressive disorder, evening primrose oil supplements may trigger an attack. Otherwise, its most famous side effect is a visible improvement in skin and hair condition.

Wild yam (Dioscorea villosa) and Mexican yam (Dioscorea mexicana)

Skin creams made from yam root are widely available at health-food shops and through the internet. They are sold as a kind of natural HRT. But although yams contain ingredients that can be converted into a form of progesterone, this has to be done in a laboratory. Creams made directly from the plant do not have hormone-like effects, and have not been found to relieve perimenopausal symptoms.

Natural progesterone

This manufactured hormone isn't a CAM remedy, though it's often mistaken for one. It's legally called 'natural' because it is made to be identical to the hormone our own bodies produce – unlike the progestogens that are more commonly used in HRT and contraceptive pills. What also seems natural, to many people, is that it's made from an ingredient found in yams. Even so, it is produced in a laboratory. Although you can buy natural progesterone on the internet, this is not recommended. Without medical tests you have no way of knowing whether your body needs this treatment and, like any drug, it can be harmful, so should not be taken without a prescription. Also, there's no control over the strength or quality of the ingredients.

Food supplements

Supplements provide vitamins, minerals and other nutrients in a much more concentrated form than you can get from food. They can be very powerful, working like medicines to tackle specific symptoms or health problems. For that reason, though, they can also have side effects, or cause a new problem to replace the one you had before. Questions have been raised about the safety and effectiveness of some once-popular supplements such as Vitamin E. Therefore it is no longer recommended that you take Vitamin E in the long term, to try to ward off diseases of old age. But, in the short term, it may help with some perimenopausal symptoms.

It's best to use supplements, especially minerals, under the guidance of a naturopath or nutritionist who has a reputable qualification and is experienced in this area. Have a consultation to find the best dose for you, and check that this is not outside the range that is considered safe. If you take any mineral supplements, take a broad-range multivitamin and mineral supplement too. Don't continue for more than three months if you're not seeing a marked improvement – and, of course, stop at once if you suffer any ill effects.

Most of the nutrients we need are available in everyday foods, especially organic produce, as long as this is fresh and minimally processed. Eating them in their natural form reduces any risk of overdosing or of causing a nutritional imbalance.

Acupuncture

There's not a lot of published evidence about the effects of acupuncture on perimenopausal symptoms, but many women say it has helped to stabilize their hormonal fluctuations. In one study, a 12-week course of acupuncture reduced flushes by 50 per cent, and the effect was still working six months later. Acupressure – working on the same points but using finger pressure instead of needles – is believed to have similar effects to acupuncture. In both cases, the effect is heavily dependent on the individual practitioner's skills, so choose with care.

Breathing your flushes away

Any kind of stress relief can ease the mental and emotional symptoms of the perimenopause, and may also reduce physical symptoms that can be triggered by stress, such as hot flushes and mood swings. Meditation is a tried-and-tested form of stress relief that costs nothing and can be done anywhere. It can be learnt in many forms.

Paced breathing works as a simple form of meditation. It has been found to reduce the number and severity of hot flushes, soothe anxiety and clear the mind. Practised every day, it will help you relax and cope more easily with any symptoms.

Start by sitting comfortably upright in a straight-backed chair with your feet on the floor. Put your hand on your stomach to feel it, rather than your upper chest, expanding as you breathe in.

Breathe in for a count of five, and then out for the same length of time. Focus on your breath, feeling it move over your upper lip as it enters and leaves your body.

When your mind wanders, bring it back to the feeling of your breath.

Practise this for ten minutes every morning and evening. Do it when you feel a hot flush about to start, as it can stop your temperature rising.

Tackling the symptoms

Insomnia

Herbal remedies that have been found to promote healthy sleep include valerian, wild lettuce and passion flower. (See later in this chapter for more on sleep and insomnia.)

Breast lumps

Evening primrose oil and chasteberry have both been found to help with breast pain and swelling or lumpiness. Many women have been helped by a 400IU Vitamin E supplement (not to be taken long term) or a Vitamin B-complex supplement containing 40–50mg Vitamin B6. (See Chapter 8 for foods that may help to combat breast pain.)

Back pain

Back pain can strike anyone in their thirties or forties, but it is often exacerbated by the menstrual irregularities of the perimenopause. Treat yourself to a new, firm mattress if your present bed is soft, but don't lie on it except at night. Try to lie on your back on the floor for 20 minutes a day, with a cushion under your knees. Staying active is important; yoga and Pilates are especially useful for the spine, but any exercise that doesn't put it under strain can help. Get an instructor, who knows you have a back problem, to show you exactly what to do, and follow the instructions. Do seek physiotherapy if back pain becomes a problem; you may be given special exercises to strengthen and support your spine.

PMS

PMS may be relieved by the same supplements recommended for breast lumps, with the addition of valerian to soothe mood swings. If you suffer premenstrual fluid retention, try vervain to stimulate the liver, motherwort to soothe menstrual pain or valerian. (See Chapter 8 for foods to combat PMS.)

Depression

For mild to moderate depression, St John's Wort has proved as effective as SSRI antidepressants, but without most of the side effects, though it has been known to increase blood pressure and interacts with some drugs. So check with your GP if you take any medicines before taking St John's Wort. Take a Vitamin B-complex supplement too, one that includes B6, B12 and folic acid. (See Chapter 3 for more help in dealing with depression.) Aerobic exercise has been proved to lift moods, so see Chapter 9 for how to get started and see also Chapter 8 for foods that fight depression.

Forgetfulness

Ginkgo biloba is better known for its effects in early dementia. But it has also been tested on healthy people, who were found to score higher marks in memory tests after taking 180mg a day. Exercise helps by improving blood supply to the brain (see Chapter 9).

Cystitis

Cranberries have the surprising effect of preventing bacteria sticking to the bladder walls. As well as drinking the juice, you can buy capsules to take in a more concentrated form. Also, dry the stalks of any organic cherries you buy and keep them in an airtight jar: a litre of hot water poured on a handful of cherry stalks, then strained and drunk when it's warm, can ease the pain of cystitis. Other remedies are uva ursi and golden seal, taken as directed. (See Chapter 8 for foods that may help.)

Thrush

Bathing your vulva in cider vinegar diluted in eight parts of water, or daubing it with plain yoghurt, can help reduce discomfort. Acidophilus capsules are said to help to re-establish healthy vaginal flora. (See Chapter 8 for tips on what to eat to reduce your risk of getting thrush.) Wear loose clothes and don't take hot baths.

Headaches

The herbal remedy feverfew has been proved to reduce the severity of headaches – some sufferers grow it in their gardens and eat the leaves in a sandwich. A study in the *British Medical Journal* in 2004 found that a short course of acupuncture could significantly reduce severe headaches and migraine. Light head massage can prevent the tightening of scalp muscles which contributes to headache.

Vitamin B6 is thought to increase resistance to pain; try it in the form of a Vitamin B-complex supplement, as B vitamins work best when combined. Fish oils may also help if you're short of these. Some naturopaths will recommend taking magnesium and calcium supplements, but it's best not to take individual mineral supplements without professional advice; try taking a daily multivitamin and multimineral tablet instead. Calcium and Vitamin D are said to work together to help prevent migraines, and our bodies make Vitamin D naturally when we're exposed to sunshine – ten minutes a day is enough. (See Chapter 8 for foods that may help.)

Constipation

Constipation is largely caused by dietary problems and a sedentary life. So the most effective natural cure is to eat more fruit and vegetables and take more exercise, especially walking or aerobics (see Chapters 8 and 9). Meanwhile, try a tablespoonful of ground linseed (flaxseed) scattered on your breakfast cereal, or the same amount of psyllium husks in a glass of warm water. Drinking plenty of warm water and eating rehydrated dried fruit can also help.

Painful joints

This perimenopausal symptom should eventually wear off by itself, unless the discomfort has made you inactive and your joints have stiffened up. To prevent this, take regular low-impact exercise: any good exercise teacher will show you the safe moves (see Chapter 9 for more details). In case it's an early sign of osteoarthritis, taking 1500mg of glucosamine sulphate a day has been proved to ease pain and slow the progress of this condition, as has 1200mg chondroitin. You could also consider using supplements of fish oil or plant oil such as evening primrose or linseed (flax seed). Antioxidant Vitamins A, C and E, plus Vitamin B-complex and zinc, may help to rebuild cartilage. (Also, see Chapter 8 for foods that may help.)

Hot flushes

To combat the vasomotor symptoms, try eating more phytoestrogens and keeping to a healthy weight – between BMI 20 and 25. (See Chapter 8 for more about eating to combat hot flushes.) Natural remedies include black cohosh, soya isoflavone supplements and possibly red clover.

Regular exercise can help your body adapt and become less sensitive to the hair-trigger changes that can launch a hot flush. If you haven't yet taken up exercise, start with something cooling such as swimming. (See Chapter 9 for more information.)

Keeping cool in all senses will reduce their frequency and strength. Hot flushes are strongly influenced by our emotions, stress and even excitement. So switch into paced-breathing mode and let your stress or anxiety seep away. Give yourself more time to get things done. Smile if it happens while you're addressing a meeting: dreading it happening simply adds to the stress, and therefore to the severity of the hot flush.

It's the same with physical heat. Wear loose layered clothes that you can easily take on and off. Carry a fan, and keep an electric fan under your desk at work. Turn the heating down: keeping to a comfortably cool level (about 19C (66F)) will reduce the pressure on your own thermostat.

Many women find their hot flushes are triggered by alcohol, coffee, spicy food or hot foods and drinks. If you've always liked your food and drinks hot, try letting them cool down a bit before you taste them.

Several studies have found that paced breathing cuts the incidence of hot flushes in half (see box). Since stress can trigger a hot flush, use any methods of stress relief that work for you.

Smoking doesn't help – smokers have more menopausal symptoms in general and hot flushes in particular.

Night sweats and insomnia

Our need for sleep drops a little during the perimenopause. Before the age of about 40, most adults need eight hours a night, whereas after that we can get by on seven. But insomnia can be one of the most annoying side effects of the perimenopause, and is often exacerbated by night sweats.

Like their daytime version, hot flushes, night sweats are caused by fluctuating hormonal levels, particularly by a sudden drop in oestrogen production. We're programmed to wake up if we get too hot, which is why light sleepers of any age are advised to turn off the bedroom radiators and not to take very hot baths in the evening. A night sweat causes such a sharp increase in temperature that you wake up suddenly, drenched, and may need to change the sheets. You may then find it hard to get back to sleep.

It is important not to fall into a pattern of sleeping badly, as insomnia can become a habit. If you're getting used to waking with night sweats and lying awake afterwards, don't soldier on. You need to restore your healthy sleeping pattern before that becomes a problem in itself. Many of the complementary therapies for perimenopause discussed in this chapter are aimed specifically at these vasomotor symptoms.

If complementary and self-help measures haven't helped within four to six weeks, and the sweats are causing you serious exhaustion and insomnia, why not consider hormone replacement therapy? Despite the question marks over its safety and efficacy in other areas, it has been proved to reduce hot flushes and night sweats – that's the one area in which its benefits outweigh the disadvantages. HRT's harmful long-term effects have mainly been found in older women who have gone through the menopause. The one group for whom it is now recommended is women who are still having periods and who suffer from troublesome vasomotor symptoms. You may need to try several formulations before finding one that controls your symptoms without causing other symptoms that irritate you even more, but it is worth persevering (see Chapter 6).

Strengthening from the inside

One of the most distressing symptoms of the perimenopause is urinary incontinence. Many women encounter this after childbirth, and if you took up pelvic-floor exercises then, you have a headstart on everyone else. Otherwise, it tends to start towards the end of the

Get a good night's sleep

If you have trouble sleeping, a few simple changes should make a difference:

- Treat yourself to a comfortable new bed with a firm mattress. Try it out by lying on it in the shop!
- Give up smoking: it has been found to cause sleep disorders including chronic insomnia.
- Take some regular daily exercise, preferably before work or at lunchtime.
- Get into the habit of going to bed and getting up at the same time every day, whether you've slept well or not.
- In the evening, don't watch action films, have arguments or do anything else that stimulates rather than helping you wind down. Even exercise can wake you up too much.
- Don't drink alcohol or have anything containing caffeine after about 6 p.m.
- Create a calming bedtime routine – for example, warm bath, peaceful music, preparing clothes for the next day – and follow it every night.
- Keep your bedroom for sleep and love-making only. Don't use it as a home office, or read anything other than a relaxing bedtime novel.
- Cut out all outside disturbances. If necessary, use earplugs and a sleep mask or blackout curtains.
- Turn down the central heating: your bedroom should be about 16–18C (60–65F) maximum.
- If you're worrying about something it's hard to let go and drop off. Write it down and resolve to deal with it tomorrow. Or, visualize your worry as a book: close it and put it in a bookshelf, telling yourself you will open it again after breakfast the next morning.
- If you've been awake more than 20 minutes, get up and do something else till you feel sleepy.

perimenopause, so taking action to strengthen the area now could prevent this happening.

As oestrogen levels wane, the bladder functions less efficiently and many women are appalled to discover that they 'leak' a few drops when they laugh or sneeze, or have such a sudden urge to urinate that they don't reach the loo in time.

A well-woman clinic can offer advice and, if necessary, help with biofeedback or devices to strengthen your internal grip. But you can get equally good results with self-help techniques.

Giving up smoking will help. Smoking robs your organs of the oxygen they need to regenerate and stay strong; its prematurely ageing effects are as damaging to internal membranes as to your complexion. Also, coughing can cause a sudden leak, and a chronic cough can weaken the muscles in the area.

The main remedy is a technique called Kegel exercises, in which you learn to tighten the muscles around the area – incidentally giving you an impressive vaginal grip! Kegel exercises have been proved to strengthen the pelvic floor, which prevents any extra pressure on the bladder. Pilates classes include a related 'zipping-up' technique that's useful to learn.

Kegel exercises are easy to do once you isolate the right muscles to work on, but this can be tricky at first, and instructions given in magazines are often misleading. Have a go with the instructions in this chapter. You may notice an improvement within a week or so. If you've tried pelvic-floor exercises on your own without success for a couple of months, ask at your doctor's surgery or well-woman clinic for help from a specially trained nurse or physiotherapist.

If you're doing weight-training, muscle-toning or aerobic exercise, it's helpful to practise Kegel exercises or the Pilates technique first. Get into the habit of holding your pelvic-floor muscles in and up before you start an exercise. Some exercises – for example, to strengthen your abdominal muscles – can push down on your pelvic floor if your posture isn't correct. Holding the pelvic floor firmly will help prevent any damage.

Kegel exercises

1 First, check you're exercising the right groups of muscles. Next time you use the loo, stop the flow of urine, let it start again and stop it again. From now on, only do this if you need to re-check that these are the muscles you're exercising. Hold in your anal muscles as if preventing yourself passing wind. Release and tighten again to get the feel of this set of muscles.

2 Slip a finger into your vagina (using a little lubricant gel if needed) and squeeze the muscles as if stopping yourself urinating. Then tighten the muscles as if to stop yourself passing wind. If

you feel your finger being gripped, you're using the right muscles. Then try to feel as if the pelvic floor is lifting itself a tiny distance up, towards your head. (*Note*: It is also possible to do this exercise without inserting a finger into the vagina. If putting a finger in your vagina is uncomfortable, rest it outside flat on the perineum, which is the skin between the vagina and the anus. If you're using the right muscles, you should feel this tiny lifting movement from the outside.)

3 Make sure you're not using other muscles. Relax your buttock muscles. Relax your thigh muscles. Relax your abdominal muscles. Don't hold your breath.

4 Ensure you're lifting muscles in and up. Rest a hand on your lower abdomen: if this pushes against your hand when you make the effort, you're straining downwards instead.

5 Hold the lift for 4 seconds, relax for 4 seconds, and repeat 10 or 15 times. Gradually work up to holding for 10 seconds at a time.

6 Do the exercises for at least 5 minutes, 3 times a day, preferably in different positions: lying, sitting and standing.

Pilates zip-up

1 Lie on your back with your knees raised and feet flat on the floor, back slightly arched.

2 Focus on the pelvic area, with your abdomen below the navel.

3 Pull the inner muscles in and up. This should bring your navel towards your spine and increase the length from ribcage to pelvis. The front of your pelvis will be slightly raised and your back will be flatter, holding its natural gentle curve.

4 Hold this inner strength as you continue your workout.

8

Eat to beat the symptoms

Study after study has revealed the effects of different micronutrients on specific conditions. Diet is now accepted as one of the most important lifestyle influences on health, capable of smoothing out hormone imbalances and perhaps even treating symptoms such as fluid retention, bloating and painful periods. It is hard to believe it can be so easy. However, putting healthy eating into practice can seem complicated. We're surrounded by a baffling range of foods in every supermarket, with more money spent on advertising new items every year.

We're also bombarded with mixed messages. From one side we hear the message that there are no good or bad foods, and everything is acceptable as part of a balanced diet. From another we're told that a third of all cancers are diet-related. Every week some new piece of research shows the benefits of certain foods, suggesting that some are indeed better than others – but which ones?

Keeping to a healthy weight is a whole minefield of its own. On the one hand we're snowed under with diet books, yet on the other we're told that fad dieting is harmful. Meanwhile we're warned that being overweight is a serious health hazard – as is being underweight.

It's not surprising if people give up in despair and just eat what they like. In fact, that's not always a bad strategy, as enjoying your food without getting stressed about it is an important part of living a happy, healthy life. And when you're young, you can get away with eating on the run or living on takeaways.

But as you leave your twenties behind, you may notice that a carefree lifestyle starts to take its toll. If you're still living the same way in your late thirties, you'll be well aware of the first effects of this: lack of energy, hangovers, minor infections that you can't shake off for weeks.

When you look at the labels on new food products, you start to notice an amazing similarity. The same cheap ingredients crop up again and again: various forms of fat, sugar, artificial sweeteners, salt and flavour-enhancing chemicals. Not really so new after all. And when you look into claims that all foods are good when eaten as part of a balanced diet, you see that they tend to come from the food industry, which would be unlikely to say anything else.

Most of us, by this stage, have discovered the joys of good food anyway. And a bonus of healthy eating is that fresh food tastes infinitely better than anything you can pick up from a takeaway or the ready-meals shelves.

'I couldn't believe how much difference it made'

Jenny, 43, had a depressing list of perimenopausal symptoms. Her periods had become so much heavier that she was taking iron tablets. She was constantly tired and irritable, suffered from constipation and headaches, and sometimes felt like running away and leaving everyone to fend for themselves. She had come to dread her work as a teacher, which she had once loved.

'It wasn't just the paperwork, which everyone hates,' she explains. 'It was the kids themselves – I couldn't cope with my own children any more, let alone a classful. I felt like screaming at them all the time.'

Her doctor did hormone tests and told her that her oestrogen level was normal. He prescribed antidepressants, which made her feel like a zombie.

'In the end it was an old friend who was really shocked by the way I ate, when she visited, and said I had to sort out my eating habits. I suddenly saw it through her eyes. I used to cook properly when I was first married, but we'd slipped into eating things the kids would eat – burgers and oven chips, pizzas. I didn't have the energy to cook separately, especially since I'd been on the antidepressants. I was eating a lot of chocolate and doughnuts during the day, and energy bars because they sounded a bit healthier.'

Spurred on by their friend, Jenny's husband started cooking proper meals when he came home from work.

'He got me to eat breakfast, which I never used to bother with,' says Jenny. 'That made a big difference straight away. I loved having dinner cooked for me, so I ate whatever he made. He even convinced me to start eating liver and cabbage, to get some more iron. Funnily, I found I quite liked it.'

She was soon feeling so much better that she gave up the iron tablets; together with the fruit and vegetables she was now eating, that was enough to cure her constipation. That in turn reduced her headaches, which were further relieved by eating regular meals instead of sweet snacks. Her job was still tiring, but she had more energy to deal with it. Eventually she weaned herself off the antidepressants.

'I went up and up,' said Jenny. 'I couldn't believe how much difference it made. My periods are still quite heavy, but I don't feel drained any more. I share the cooking now – I still don't like cooking so I use a lot of frozen veg, but that's fine. I'm not tempted to miss a meal or eat doughnuts any more, because if I do I feel exhausted before the end of the day.'

Perimenopausal changes and digestion

The hormonal changes of the perimenopause have surprisingly strong effects on the digestive system. First, you may take longer to feel comfortably full when you're eating; naturally, this encourages you to eat more. This is because a drop in oestrogen production slows down the working of the gall-bladder, which is supposed to send you a signal when you've eaten enough. And, although you may not feel full, your stomach is actually taking longer to empty.

If these two changes are happening at the same time, as they often do, you risk suffering both indigestion and weight gain. Serve meals on a smaller plate, eat slowly, and don't prepare enough to have second helpings. If you're still hungry, wait for ten minutes before eating more, as it sometimes takes this long for fullness to register.

Also, changes in insulin metabolism may be making your body turn carbohydrates into fat instead of using them for ready energy. To counteract this, eat small, regular meals that combine protein and a small amount of fat with vegetables, salad or wholemeal grains.

Acid reflux is another possible problem, as progesterone relaxes the muscle that normally stops acid flowing up out of the stomach. Eating hot, spicy meals may lead to acid pains in the chest and throat, especially if you eat late in the evening and lie down soon after. Keep spicy foods for lunchtime, or eat dinner a little earlier.

As digestion becomes less efficient and partly digested food moves through to the intestines, bloating and wind also become a problem. Sugar and fatty foods are most likely to cause wind by fermenting, so cut down on them.

Gallstones become more likely, and can build up to dangerous levels before making themselves felt with bouts of pain. Cut down your risk by reducing your intake of saturated fats.

Hormonal changes also reduce the efficiency of the bowel, leading to constipation, which in turn increases the risk of other unwelcome changes such as varicose veins. Prevent this by being physically active, especially by regularly walking or running. Eat plenty of natural fibre: not bran, but high-fibre foods such as fresh fruit, vegetables and wholegrain cereals. Also, ensure you drink plenty of fluid.

What are the best choices?

Decades of research have confirmed that the food group almost everyone needs most is fruit and vegetables. While not enough, alone, to meet all our needs, they provide more nutrition than anything else you can eat. As well as fruit and vegetables, which provide the best form of carbohydrate along with an alphabet of vitamins and other nutrients, you need some starchy foods to fill up on. Bread, pasta and rice meet this need, along with potatoes, the starchiest vegetable.

Fat is a necessary part of our diet – so necessary in fact that we evolved with a taste for it to ensure that we'd always make an effort to find some. Without any fat in our diet, we would not be able to use some of the other nutrients from food. But fat today is such a cheap ingredient that processed foods are stuffed full of it, and its pleasing taste and texture keep calling us back for more. However, fats used in processed foods are often in hydrogenated form, which has question marks over its safety. A healthier way of getting the fat we need is from nut or vegetable oils and from oily fish.

Protein is another need that modern diets meet all too adequately. We do need high-protein foods such as meat, fish, dairy, eggs, beancurd or vegetarian meat substitutes, but it's often sold in forms that include unwelcome ingredients. Fast foods such as burgers may be made of animal parts you wouldn't want to eat, as well as laden with fat. The less processed a food is when you buy it, the more control you have over what you're eating. Organic meat and dairy produce are the healthiest protein choices, along with organic soya products such as beancurd.

Why eat organic?

To keep the price down, industrially produced meat is raised under intensive conditions, with routine use of drugs to prevent the diseases that these cause or to promote growth. A lot of meat, especially made into cheap products, contains drug and chemical residues. Chicken is popular as a cheap low-fat option, but is frequently found to contain food-poisoning bacteria. Fruit and vegetables, especially salad leaves, are routinely found to contain residues of pesticides, including some that have been banned for many years.

Genetically modified (GM) food is another industrial innovation that many people are wary of. The first GM crop was soya beans, modified to resist a specific pesticide produced by the same company. Because the pesticide killed all other plant life except the soya beans, farmers used it in large quantities. Since then, other crops have been bred with different traits, all offering some benefit to industrial-scale producers.

Smaller-scale farmers were concerned about modified genes spreading, breeding superweeds and having unknown effects on other plant life. Environmentalists complained that overuse of pesticides damaged the soil and put more residues on food and into the water supply. Conservationists noted that arid fields of GM crops reduced the habitat for butterflies and other animal life. Medics were concerned that the genes in some GM crops could spread resistance to antibiotics – a growing problem in hospitals around the world. Recent studies have also started to raise questions about possible health risks from GM foods.

As the GM foods offer no benefit to consumers, people have been reluctant to buy them. But the powerful US agrochemical industry has been successful in countering some European legislation designed to keep food GM-free, or at least to have it clearly labelled. Soya is the largest GM crop, along with the cereal that's called maize in the UK and corn in the USA, and these are contained in many processed foods. So it's not always possible to be certain that processed foods are GM-free.

Organic food is pretty much immune to these problems. The fruit and vegetables are grown without artificial chemicals, so there is no risk of residues either on the skin or throughout the plant. Organic animals are not dosed with drugs or artificial hormones; they are only given medicines as needed if they are ill, and are not slaughtered until the residues have left their bodies. They only eat natural foodstuffs and, as a result, no organically raised cattle ever had mad-cow disease during the epidemic of the 1980s and 1990s (the very few cases found in organic herds were in animals that had been bought in). And organic food is not allowed to contain GM ingredients or hydrogenated fats (see Chapter 10).

This traditional kind of farming isn't just good for our own health – it's also good for animals and for the environment. Organic farmers aren't allowed to exhaust the soil with artificial fertilizers or kill everything they can't sell with poisons that seep into the ground and into our water supply. By law, any food sold as organic has to meet levels of animal welfare way above those allowed in standard intensive farming – and much of the cheap meat eaten in the UK is imported from countries with even less animal protection than here.

Organic food used to be the province of people who either grew their own or paid a premium to buy succulent, knobbly vegetables from small specialist farm shops. But even supermarkets now have a wide range of organic items. Box-delivery schemes, easily found on the internet or through the Soil Association (see Useful addresses), keep prices down and quality high.

If you can afford it, organic is an excellent investment in your own health and the environment. Most of us, though, need to weigh up quality against price. In this case, you need to choose the organic items that are generally most intensively farmed, or are most likely to contain GM ingredients, or that could do most harm if contaminated in any way.

For this reason, the most important items to buy organic are:

- Meat (especially beef and poultry).
- Dairy produce.
- Soya products such as beancurd and many vegetarian products; soya is also found in many fast foods, but there's no way of checking this before you buy.
- Salad leaves: avoid non-organic ready-washed salads in particular, as they're likely to have been washed in chlorine.
- Broccoli, cabbages and other leafy vegetables.
- Carrots – or cut the first 3cm (a good inch) off the tops if they're non-organic.
- Anything that's bought out of season. Or try growing your own vegetables – if you've no garden, a growbag will provide three or four tomato plants, some beet spinach or some beetroot (all very easy to grow).

Your lifelong health and vitality diet

This healthy-eating plan is quite low in fat and very low in the simple carbohydrates that add calories without nutrition. It's largely based on foods that are low on the glycaemic index (GI), meaning that they provide long-lasting energy rather than making your blood-sugar level suddenly surge then fall again. This means it's filling and nutritious, reducing your urge to eat unhealthy snacks. If you're overweight, it will help you lose weight at a steady pace. If you're underweight, you can use it to gain weight healthily.

You don't need to throw out everything you usually eat and start again. If you currently eat a standard Western diet based on processed foods, just incorporating some of these principles will bring about major improvements. The most important change is to eat more fruit and vegetables, so make that your first step: adding a couple of servings of vegetables or salad to every meal and replacing bought snacks with fruit.

Vegetables are the basis of a healthy diet. There are literally hundreds to choose from, so branch out and try some new tastes. This is one food group most of us can safely eat in unlimited amounts. Aim for at least five servings a day of vegetables – more is better. Don't eat more than one serving of potatoes a day, as these are high-GI.

Fruit is almost as nutritious as vegetables, so aim for at least three servings a day. Fresh is best, but tinned fruit in juice is fine, as is dried fruit soaked in water. Being sweeter than vegetables, fruits are usually higher in calories, but are still far less fattening than practically any other sweet foods. If you're trying to lose weight, don't eat more than three servings a day, and avoid dried fruit.

Fill up with good-quality starchy foods too: granary bread, wholegrain cereals, non-instant rice and pasta. Avoid the white versions of all these. Two or three servings a day are recommended.

Try adding some nuts, seeds and legumes to your diet. They make a healthy snack, and are also the basis of good oils such as sunflower. Have one to three servings a day, or a little less if you're trying to lose weight.

Eat one or two servings a day of organic meat, fish, eggs and other high-protein foods, including oily fish at least twice a week.

Dairy foods are full of bone-strengthening calcium in a form our bodies easily absorb. One or two servings a day are recommended, preferably low-fat. If you love full-fat cheese but need to watch your weight or cholesterol levels, just eat it in smaller amounts.

The smallest section includes white flour and sweet products such as sugar, cakes and biscuits. Much as we love these sweet tastes, they're unnecessary and are harmful to health if eaten more often than as the occasional treat. Try not to eat more than one serving of these a day. Alcohol falls into the same category – preferably only one unit of it a day.

If your weight isn't a problem, there's no harm in enjoying cakes and desserts made with natural ingredients such as wholemeal cereals and fruit. If buying rather than making these, make sure they're not full of sugar in various forms, including honey, fructose and other ingredients ending in '-ose'. Diet or 'lite' products are low in sugar, but a glance at the label will usually reveal that they're full of unhealthy additives, especially artificial sweeteners. These have been linked with various health risks, including cancer.

Rules of thumb

A 'serving', as defined by the World Health Organization, is 80g (nearly 3oz). For most foods, that's roughly as much as you can hold in one hand.

Meat and fish: a piece as big and thick as the palm of your hand.
Bread rolls: the size of your fist.
Bread: one slice.
Cheese: a 2.5cm (1in) cube, about the size of the top joint of your thumb.
Pasta: a bundle of dry spaghetti 2.5cm (1in) across, or two fistfuls of cooked pasta.
Pasta sauce: a ladleful as big as your fist.
Fruit juice: a 150ml glass.
Berry-sized fruit: one small bowl of strawberries, grapes, etc.
Small fruit: two plums, satsumas, etc.
Medium-sized fruit: one apple, pear, etc.
Large fruit: one big slice of melon, etc.
Cooked fruit and vegetables: 2 to 3 tablespoonfuls.
Beans and pulses: 2 tablespoonfuls.
Salad: one small mixed side salad.
Dried fruit, nuts and seeds: about a handful.
Oils and fats: a teaspoonful.

Staying in shape

Starting from the mid-thirties, most women gain an average of $\frac{1}{2}$–1kg (1–2lb) a year in weight. This is partly because of hormonal changes leading up to the menopause. It doesn't sound like much and, at first, it's imperceptible.

But if you don't do anything to prevent this, you'll wake up in your fifties to find yourself weighed down by anything up to 20kg (3 stone) of fat that has become very hard to shift. Much of it will be around your stomach area, increasing your risk of heart disease. And nothing makes you look more middle-aged than that solid bulk round your middle!

It's best to take action as soon as you start straying beyond the limits of a healthy weight range. That doesn't mean decades of self-deprivation in an effort to keep to your youthful dress size all your life. Unrealistic goals put you under needless stress. Anyway, thinness carries its own health risks as you get older, osteoporosis being the main one. But you've a better chance of staying fit and healthy if you keep to a body-mass index (BMI) of about 20 to 25.

If you do need to lose weight, it's important to do it before you reach the menopause. After that time, it's much more difficult to lose weight: hormonal changes make your body cling to every kilo. Early in the perimenopause, even when your hormones have started changing, they're still at levels that make it relatively easy to lose weight and to maintain, or regain, the shape you'd like to keep.

Start by checking your BMI (see box) to see if you're a healthy weight for your height. If it's above 30, you should have a health check-up and ask your GP if there's a local group or other facilities to help you lose weight.

Although most weight-loss products are a waste of money, some studies published in nutrition journals suggest that adding cayenne pepper, tabasco sauce or ginger to your food will help you feel full sooner and possibly even increase your metabolism by a small amount. Green tea is also said to help you burn calories faster – and since it's also hailed for its health-enhancing qualities, you've nothing to lose by drinking it.

The safest and easiest way to lose weight is not to go on a diet, but to take up healthier eating habits. This should allow you to lose 1–2kg a month (depending on how overweight you are) without really noticing. The healthy-eating programme above should help you stay at a healthy weight, and lose any extra. If you find you're not losing weight on the healthy-eating plan, and your BMI is over 25, swap to the lower-calorie version until your weight settles at a healthy level.

Why are you putting on weight?

The hormonal changes of the perimenopause blunt our body's signals that we've eaten enough, and turn carbohydrates more readily into fat. Luckily, hormones aren't the only cause of weight gain in the forties, and we have more control over the other factors.

One main reason for putting on weight is that we become less physically active while still eating the same amount. Simply leaving the car in the garage can help.

If you have children, you may end up eating the kind of fatty, sugary foods that appeal to them – and possibly finishing off their meals to prevent waste. (Remember you're not a waste-disposal unit!) The junk-food diet most children choose if they have a chance is manufactured to appeal to their unsophisticated tastes, but it's as unhealthy for them as it is for you. It has been linked with poor school results, lethargy and aggression as well as physical diseases.

It may be hard to get children to eat healthy food, but it's not impossible: numerous cookbooks, magazine features and television programmes can help with ideas. Or read *Help Your Child Get Fit Not Fat* by Jan Hurst and Sue Hubberstey (see Further reading). Families who sit down to eat together tend to have healthier food and fewer weight problems. So eat together round a table, without snacks available as a back-up for those who don't want to join in. You could be startled by the improvement in the children's well-being as well as your own. Even just increasing the number of vegetables you serve will make a big difference to the whole family's health.

Statistics show that women over 30 are drinking more alcohol than ever before, wreaking havoc on their shape as well as their general health. It's not only full of empty calories: alcohol can actually affect women's hormones enough to cause male patterns of weight gain, with fat building up on the stomach and abdomen.

Emotional upheaval or PMS push many of us into comfort-eating. It's certainly a better 'comforter' than, say, alcohol, but it's a vicious circle if an expanding waistline makes you even more depressed. (See Chapter 3 for help that doesn't harm.)

Meanwhile, soothe your sweet tooth with fruit instead of cakes or bought desserts that may give you a brief lift, but leave you feeling more tired and empty than before. Fruit, on the other hand, boosts your vitality, makes your skin glow and is packed with fibre and nutrients. If you're trying to lose weight, don't eat unlimited fruit – three servings a day is a good amount.

Two-thirds of the British population is now overweight or obese – we're the eighth fattest nation in the world. This is partly because we're all cooking less and eating more manufactured food, bulked up with cheap and fattening fillers. But it's also because portion sizes have ballooned: from bars of chocolate to fast-food meals, every-thing has expanded in size to tempt us with ever-more enormous bargains. Why are the manufacturers so generous? Because the ingredients are the cheapest part of the operation for them. Special offers also tempt us to buy more products in larger quantities than we'd intended: if we buy three for the price of two, we're still spending extra, especially if it is a product we wouldn't usually buy.

We've become so used to supersized food when we eat out that we've started serving larger portions at home too. One portion, or serving, of any food should weigh about 80g (just under 3oz). To get a feeling for portion size, try weighing all your food for a week or two – you may be surprised. Cutting down to what used to be normal portion sizes could leave you feeling hungry at first, but that's a chance to meet two health targets in one: fill the gaps by piling on plenty of extra vegetables to get at least five servings a day.

Find your BMI

Divide your weight in kilograms (kg) by the square of your height in metres (m). So if you're 1.65m tall and weigh 57kg, your BMI is 57 divided by (1.65 x 1.65 =) 2.72, which comes to just under 21.

Or multiply your weight in pounds by 700 and divide it by the square of your height in inches. If you're 5ft 5in tall and weigh 9 stone, or 126 pounds, that's (126 x 700 =) 88,200, divided by (65 x 65 =) 4,225, which comes to just under 21.

Or do it online at www.bbc.co.uk/health/healthy_living/your _weight/bmiimperial_index.shtml.

A BMI under 19 is considered to be underweight, over 25 is overweight, and over 30 is obese. Between 19 and 25 is healthy.

Eat to solve perimenopausal symptoms

Some foods offer particular benefits for specific health problems, so try adding them to your diet for a few weeks. They shouldn't affect any medicine or complementary remedies you're taking, but check with your doctor or pharmacist just in case.

If you suspect that food is playing a role in your symptoms, keep a diary and note everything (including sweets and snacks) you've eaten and drunk each day, with the time you had them. Also note what symptoms you have and when. Keep this diary for at least a month and see if any patterns emerge.

As with any self-help measures, if these don't help within six to twelve weeks, and the symptom is troubling you, see your GP.

Hot flushes and night sweats

Phytoestrogens are the best-known dietary answer to the vasomotor symptoms (see Chapter 7 for information about taking them in the form of supplements). Soya is the most popular source of phytoestrogens for women seeking relief from hot flushes. Soya-based foods such as beancurd (tofu), tempeh and miso are high in protein too, so they're a useful alternative to meat. Stir-frying vegetables with beancurd and soya sauce produces a quick and tasty meal that's packed with nutrients. Soya foods are often made from GM beans unless otherwise stated, so buy organic to be sure.

Three or four servings of phytoestrogen-rich food a day have been found to reduce many women's hot flushes considerably. The Women's Nutritional Advisory Service recommends about 100mg of isoflavones a day to control severe hot flushes, eaten in small quantities throughout the day. As a rough guide, you will find approximately 20mg of isoflavones in a 250ml glass of soya milk, approximately 12mg in a soya yogurt or dessert, 25mg in 100g of tofu, and 8mg in a tablespoon of organic golden linseeds (flax seeds). Linseeds are almost as high in phytoestrogens as soya, so add some to your breakfast cereals and look out for linseed bread in the shops.

Eat small, regular meals with plenty of vegetables. A low-fat diet has been found to reduce the frequency of hot flushes over a long period.

Have at least one serving of high-protein food and two a day of dairy foods, including semi-skimmed milk.

Fast food and empty-calorie snacks reduce your nutritional status and increase hormonal imbalances.

Mood swings and depression

If you can feel your temper fraying as you become hungry, organize regular small meals interspersed with wholesome snacks. Try to avoid sugary comfort foods, which unbalance your blood-sugar levels still further.

The amino acid phenylalanine helps prevent depression; get plenty of it in protein-rich foods such as milk, cheese, meat and fish. Foods rich in the B vitamins help too (see PMS below). Although the artificial sweetener aspartame also contains a source of phenylalanine, this form has never been linked with any benefits to health or mood, and there are safety question marks over the use of aspartame.

Tiredness

Fatigue is one of the clearest signs of poor nutrition. It is also one of the easiest to cure, by switching to healthier eating patterns, with regular meals (including breakfast) and more fruit and vegetables.

Eat a high-protein, low-fat lunch if you tend to feel lethargic in the early afternoon. Good options are meat or beancurd and steamed vegetables if you're cooking. For a packed lunch, take ham or cottage cheese with plenty of salad. Don't drink alcohol at lunchtime.

Daytime tiredness is often caused by poor sleeping patterns. Carbohydrates encourage sleep, so have pasta, baked potato or thick soup and a roll for your evening meal. Other foods that promote sleep include milk (a hot milky drink is a traditional night-cap) and bananas.

Headaches and migraine

Most migraine sufferers know that certain foods will trigger their shattering pain, and ordinary headaches may also be caused this way. You may discover that you only need to avoid your danger foods during or just before a period.

If missing a meal triggers a headache, or if you rely on snacks and fast food during the day, low blood sugar may be a culprit. Eat regular meals with healthy snacks in between.

If you have regular attacks, try leaving out foods from the following 'trigger' list for two weeks and, if you stay pain-free, start reintroducing them to your diet until you discover which ones cause an attack. Common culprits are chocolate, cheese and dairy produce, citrus fruits, alcohol, fried foods, nuts, meat, wheat, tomatoes, onions, corn, apples, bananas or the sweetener aspartame. Many sufferers are sensitive to tyramine, found in sour or fermented goods such as aged cheeses, pickled herrings, soya sauce and beer. Try to cut down on saturated fat to improve circulation.

Ginger can ease the pain of headaches and migraine. Brown rice, cooked green or leafy vegetables and non-citrus fruits are unlikely to cause headaches in anyone, and beans contain masses of migraine-fighting calcium. Whole grains, dried non-citrus fruits, broccoli and spinach are rich in magnesium, which in several studies has proved effective in treating or easing migraine and premenstrual headaches.

Coffee is an odd substance because, though some people find it triggers a migraine, others say that two strong cups at the start of an attack can ward it off.

Digestive disorders

These take many forms, but heartburn and constipation are among the commonest during the perimenopause.

Eating plenty of fresh fruit and vegetables will prevent constipation and reduce the risk of irritable bowel syndrome, which can lead on from chronic constipation. Non-instant rice and oats are also recommended. Eat ginger, in any form you like, to prevent nausea – it's been proved more effective than standard anti-nausea drugs. Drink peppermint tea to improve digestion unless you suffer from heartburn, which it may exacerbate. Liquorice has been found to protect the stomach lining.

If you eat a lot of raw fruit and vegetables, this may be what's irritating your stomach. Try eating more cooked food to see if that helps. If hot food causes stomach ache, let it cool down to room temperature.

Avoid coffee and alcohol, which irritate the digestive tract. Fatty foods, chocolate and tomatoes also increase the risk of digestive problems.

Menstrual problems: pain, PMS and heavy bleeding

Like many other perimenopausal symptoms, period pains and PMS can be eased by eating foods that balance the hormones. Don't comfort-eat the sort of rich foods that we all crave during hormonal swings. A low-fat diet has been found to help many women with menstrual problems. Increasing your fibre intake from fruit and vegetables may help to control hormone metabolism. Eat a diet rich in essential fatty acids, especially fish oils, which have anti-inflammatory properties.

Painful periods are often linked with a shortage of magnesium, so magnesium-rich foods such as peanuts, Brazil nuts, almonds, muesli, oatmeal, dried fruit and dried skimmed milk may help.

If you're bleeding heavily, it's important to eat enough iron-rich food to prevent anaemia. Heavy periods leave you short of iron, but this shortage can then make your periods even heavier, so do visit your doctor to get this sorted out. If you're anaemic, you may be prescribed iron supplements (don't take them without a prescription), but these often cause constipation; those in liquid form are said to be less constipating.

Even if an anaemia test is negative, your iron stores may be low – about a tenth of all women are thought to fall into this category – so it's worth eating to increase your iron stores as long as you are still having periods. Choose foods rich in both iron and Vitamin C, which helps your body to absorb iron. The best iron sources are from animal foods: red meat, liver, fish and eggs. So vegetarians should consider taking a simple daily multivitamin and multimineral supplement. Also, add kidney beans, salad leaves, dark green vegetables and fruit, especially citrus fruits.

Research by the Women's Nutritional Advisory Service has found that different types of PMS respond to different foods. For all forms of PMS, they've discovered, you need more Vitamin B6 and magnesium – these alone could cure mood swings and tension. For more Vitamin B6, eat fish, liver, bacon, beans, Marmite, tomato puree and bananas. There's both magnesium and Vitamin B6 in wholemeal bread, soya flour, mung beans and nuts.

If you feel bloated, with tender breasts, extra Vitamin E is recommended, from salmon, tuna, oils (sunflower-seed, peanut, olive or cod-liver), nuts, blackberries, spinach and avocado. For PMS headaches, tiredness and craving for sweets: add chromium from rye bread, calf liver, eggs, brewer's yeast, peppers and potatoes. If it takes the form of depression, confusion and insomnia: try Vitamin C from blackcurrants, parsley, canned guavas, strawberries, peppers, raw red cabbage and of course oranges.

Other researchers have found calcium helpful. And one survey of 3,000 women, published in the *Archives of Internal Medicine* in 2005, showed that PMS was significantly less of a problem among those whose diets were rich in both calcium and Vitamin D. So make sure you're getting enough calcium from salmon, beancurd (tofu), dried fruit, nuts and green leafy vegetables, and Vitamin D from fish, liver or eggs. Fizzy soft drinks rob your bones of calcium; have a drink of milk instead. Eating meat more than once a day may reduce your body's ability to use calcium. Bran and other foods with laxative effects can rush food through your system so fast that you don't have time to absorb all the nutrients, so don't use these unless you have to.

One of the best sources for both calcium and Vitamin D is low-fat dairy produce, and you can also get both from wholegrain cereals and broccoli. The body also makes Vitamin D from sunlight on the skin – yet another reason to go out for a walk or a run any time when you're not at risk of getting sunburnt.

Fluid retention and swollen breasts

Salt increases fluid retention, so cut down on salty foods. Sugar may also be linked with fluid retention, so try to avoid this too. Eat as little processed food as possible, since most of our salt and sugar intake is hidden in these. Try to drink water or fruit juice instead of coffee, tea and soft drinks.

Do get plenty of potassium from fruit and vegetables, meat, fish, beans and rice. Have plenty of green vegetables or salad daily.

Cystitis and thrush

Avoid spicy, greasy, salty or acidic foods, which can predispose you to these infections. Sugary foods feed both these irritating disorders, so as soon as you notice the first signs, cut down on all sweet foods – not just snacks and alcohol, but even sweet fruit juice. Cranberry juice is the one exception: it stops bacteria taking hold, so drink plenty of this, even if it's sweetened. Drink all the water you can swallow when you're having a cystitis attack, to dilute the burning pain.

Muscle pains

In many people, symptoms are triggered by the same foods that cause migraines, so try the anti-migraine measures given above. Cut down on high-fat foods and check your food diary to detect any other triggers: some people's muscle pain has been found to be triggered by a reaction to food preservatives, monosodium glutamate, caffeine, food colourings, chocolate, shrimps or dairy products.

Eat plenty of high-carbohydrate foods such as wholemeal bread, pasta, potatoes and fruit to increase the brain's production of the natural painkiller serotonin – people suffering chronic pain for no obvious reason are often low in this.

Some complementary practitioners recommend a low-fat vegan diet. But if you cut out all animal produce including eggs and dairy, you need to eat very carefully and take supplements to ensure you have enough nutrients.

Occasionally muscle pain can be linked to low blood pressure, so get your GP to check that yours is in the normal range.

Painful joints

This is one of the most unexpected symptoms of the perimenopause, and doesn't always wear off after your periods stop. By restricting your mobility, it can increase the risk of long-term pain. Luckily, it's one of the areas in which dietary therapies claim most success.

Do eat plenty of oily fish such as sardines, mackerel and salmon, since these are rich in the fatty acids that counteract inflammation. A diet high in vegetables and oats should keep the bowel working efficiently, reducing the risk of anything harmful lingering in the body. Fruit and vegetables provide Vitamin C and other nutrients that help repair damaged joints. Red or orange fruit and vegetables are rich in helpful carotenoids. Green vegetables, beans and fruit are rich in alpha-linolenic acid (ALA), which fights inflammation.

Don't eat a lot of meat. Organic chicken with the skin removed has least of the animal fats that promote inflammation. Naturopaths believe that plants from the nightshade family (tomatoes, potatoes, aubergines and peppers) also promote inflammation, so try cutting these out for a few weeks to see if your pain eases.

9

The fitness solution

Because your metabolism starts to slow down in your thirties, making it easier to gain weight, and harder to lose it, one of the most attractive benefits of exercise at this stage is that it can shake off the excess pounds and even speed your metabolism up a little. Now is the time to do it, because hormonal changes make it much more difficult to lose excess weight later in the perimenopause.

Other beneficial changes from exercise include glowing skin, a sign of improved blood circulation, and an increase in energy to counteract the fatigue that so many women notice as an early sign of perimenopause. Increased fitness can even reduce perimenopausal mood swings.

This is also a good time to work on your posture. Backache, common in perimenopause, is exacerbated by long-term poor posture and a sedentary life. Improving your fitness now helps to keep your back strong and flexible, and to strengthen your abdominal muscles to support your spine.

Flexibility too is vital to reduce joint and muscle symptoms during the perimenopause and is easier to build up in your thirties than when you're near the menopause.

Any fitness improvements you make now will keep repaying you through the rest of your life, starting with your experience of the perimenopause. A nightmare of mood swings, niggling pain and hot flushes, or just another life-stage with as many ups as downs? You have more control over that than you may think.

Keeping it is easier than getting it back

Up to their forties, fitness is relatively easy for women to achieve, simple to maintain, and not too hard to regain (with a bit of effort) if you lose it. From your forties onwards, fitness is harder to gain and easier to lose – but, if you build it into your lifestyle, it is fairly easy to maintain.

Workout for your hormones

Regular exercise works in several ways to ease the perimenopausal transition. Individual symptoms can be alleviated by certain types of exercise.

More generally, your cells need oxygen in order to function, so increasing their oxygen supply helps your whole system to work better. Because aerobic, or cardiovascular, exercise improves the heart's ability to pump oxygen-rich blood around the body, your all-round health improves.

And there's some evidence that exercise itself may regulate the production of hormones. Any lively movement that you enjoy can create a rush of 'feel-good' endorphins, for example, whether it's dancing the tango, taking an aerobics class or making love.

Aerobic exercise – the sort that raises your heart rate, such as walking fast or doing a step class – is believed to have a moderating effect on the reproductive hormones that fluctuate during the perimenopause. For this reason, some women find that regular aerobic exercise eases the vasomotor symptoms: hot flushes and night sweats.

If you are already getting these symptoms, which react badly to an increase in temperature, you won't want to do a workout that brings you out in a sweat. In this case, swimming is an ideal aerobic exercise with a built-in cooling factor.

Yoga is also claimed to have beneficial effects on hormones, especially the forward bends, which are said to stimulate the endocrine system and the reproductive organs.

Symptomatic relief through exercise

There's some evidence that regular aerobic exercise can regulate the *menstrual cycle*. If you're bleeding heavily, though, do gentle stretching exercises instead to avoid increasing the flow. These can ease period pain and associated backache. Then continue with the aerobic exercise between periods.

One symptom that many women don't realize is hormonal is *joint pain*. A lot of women develop niggling aches, which they trace back to some over-enthusiastic DIY or carrying a heavy four-year-old home from the park, and wonder why it hasn't worn off. This kind of minor injury or overuse can, of course, lead to joint or muscle pain. But hormonal changes can also make your joints ache at this time of life, without any other trigger.

If you have pain in the joints, first get your doctor to check there isn't some other cause, such as arthritis (which can strike at any age) or injury. If this isn't the case, don't try to protect the joints by cutting back on exercise. It's important to stay active for two reasons: exercise can help regulate the hormones that cause the pain, and inactivity makes joints stiffen up.

Do gentle stretching exercises to keep joints and muscles mobile, with some muscle-building work to support them: Pilates provides a good combination. Yoga is another valuable option, as long as the teacher knows your problem and helps you avoid putting pressure on your joints.

With luck, working on flexibility and posture in your thirties should prevent joint pain taking hold. It can affect anyone during the perimenopause, as it depends to some extent on hormonal levels, but is a lot more likely to hit women who lead sedentary lives.

Related to this is the *clumsiness* that suddenly strikes many women during the perimenopause. It's startling and distressing to feel like a bull in a china shop, dropping coffee mugs and risking the safety of any child within collision range.

This loss of balance and co-ordination is one of the disorienting symptoms that take many women by surprise. Because it's linked with the hormonal fluctuations of the perimenopause, it should ease off eventually. But as with joint and muscle pain, limiting your activity will prevent recovery, so counteract it with exercises that improve balance and co-ordination. The standing yoga poses and qi gong are excellent for balance. To improve co-ordination, if you're feeling energetic, try football practice – keeping the ball in the air – or juggling, or even a dance-mat machine. Tai chi is good for both balance and co-ordination.

Insomnia during the perimenopause may or may not be hormone-related. But as with joint pain, the right kind of exercise can relieve it whatever the cause. Sleeping patterns are improved by regular aerobic exercise, preferably in the morning or early evening, as some people find it wakes them up too much at night. Slow, meditative exercise such as tai chi is excellent in the evening, to stop your mind racing.

For many women, hormonal changes cause *constipation*, a perimenopausal nightmare of headaches, discomfort and unwellness, that can lead on to irritable bowel syndrome (IBS) and varicose veins. Luckily, constipation is one of the easiest symptoms to control, with a change of diet and a more active lifestyle. The body needs a certain amount of everyday movement to keep it function-ing, which is why constipation is also common among people who lead a very sedentary life. Often, just being more active is enough to solve the problem: walking instead of taking the car or bus for short journeys; striding upstairs instead of waiting for a lift; shopping in the market or high street instead of ordering food online. If that's not enough (combined with the dietary changes suggested in Chapter 8), take up regular aerobic exercise, including a brisk walk or a run every day. Borrow a neighbour's dog, if you haven't got one of your own, and take it for long walks in the park.

Finally, *emotional disturbances* such as depression, anxiety and mood swings are very distressing symptoms of the perimenopause. Aerobic exercise is one of the most effective treatments for these – not only in helping to smooth out the hormonal roller-coaster, but also in raising self-esteem and well-being.

One study of more than 200 perimenopausal women found that those who led active lives had significantly fewer and less distressing psychological and sexual symptoms than inactive women of the same age. The active women were much less likely to be irritable or forgetful or lose their libido; also, they suffered fewer headaches and less vaginal dryness.

Yoga is calming and helps to restore a feeling of control. In addition to any effect it may have on the hormones, it alleviates many symptoms by reducing tension and improving flexibility and co-ordination. Yoga teachers often recommend forward-bends to relieve anxiety, supported back-bends for fatigue, and chest-opening positions to lift the spirits.

Body audit

If you have a long mirror at home, or next time you're trying on clothes in a shop, take a few minutes while undressed to have a good objective look at your body – not to find fault with it, but to see how you can keep it in the best possible shape.

Check your natural posture from all angles – make a point of standing normally, not trying to be straighter than usual. Is one shoulder or hip higher or further forward than the other? Is your back slumped or your waist excessively arched? Is your head bowed or your chin jutting? Do your feet turn in or out? Are you slightly knock-kneed or bow-legged?

All of these can be signs of damage to your spine or just bad posture, which can cause pain and unfitness if you don't straighten them out. The pattern of wear on your shoe soles can tell you more about this. Or step on to a bath mat with wet feet and see if the imprint of your feet is uneven in any way.

Postural problems are some of the easiest to correct, and in the most rewarding way: you immediately start to look taller, slimmer and more graceful. You can see the difference so quickly that you'll be highly motivated to continue. And you're not just looking better – you're helping to prevent a surprisingly long list of disorders from backache to heart disease.

What about your weight and shape? Are your abdominal muscles very weak? Is your skin starting to look a bit slack, suggesting that the underlying muscle tone is poor? You've probably already noticed if you have the dimpled fat known as cellulite on your hips and thighs. But is it visible anywhere else? Are you pot-bellied or generally overweight? Or are you painfully thin?

For these, you need to work on your muscles. Weight-training or other forms of muscle-toning exercise will firm you up, and improve your shape if you're too skinny. If you're overweight, you'll need to do enough aerobic exercise to burn off some fat. If you're either overweight or underweight, a healthy-eating programme is also important.

Again, the immediate benefits are to your looks, but the long-term results are also beneficial to your health. Excess weight can predispose you to heart disease, diabetes and some cancers; it's also an obstacle to getting fit. If you're underweight, you're at risk of osteoporosis and infertility, and you may suffer more from certain perimenopausal symptoms such as the dreaded hot flushes.

Back up this visual check by testing your cardiovascular fitness – how well your heart is working. When did you last run for a bus or walk upstairs rather than taking the lift or the escalator? If that wasn't recently, you can be fairly sure you aren't as fit as you thought. Try the step test (see box) or, for a very rough fitness test, time yourself walking so fast that you're almost breaking into a run. If you're glad to stop at the end of a minute, you'd better get down to the gym.

As part of your fitness audit, consider what your genetic tendencies hold in store (see Chapter 10 for clues on what action to take now).

Fit for anything

The main elements of any fitness programme will be aerobic exercise, muscle-building or toning, and flexibility.

The step test

To find out how fit you are, do this test, based on one devised by the Canadian Public Health Association. You'll need a watch with a second hand and a 30cm/12in step. Any gym will have steps made for exercise, or just use the bottom step of a staircase. Check before you start that you know how to find your pulse, either at the front of your wrist or on the side of your neck.

Start by stepping up with the right foot, then the left foot, so you're standing on the step. Then down with the right foot, then with the left foot, so you're standing on the floor again. Put your whole foot down at every step – don't do it on your toes.

Timing yourself, step up and down steadily for 3 minutes, aiming to go up and down twice in 5 seconds, or 24 times a minute. Keep to a steady 4-beat cycle by saying 'up, up, down, down' as you step.

Take your pulse for a minute as soon as you've finished. The slower it is, the more fit you are.

For a woman aged 36 to 45, a heart rate of:

- 90 or less is excellent,
- 102 is good,
- 103–110 is better than average,
- 111–118 is average,
- 119–128 is below average,
- 129–140 is poor,
- more than 140 is very poor.

If you're aged 26 to 35, your pulse rate should be a few beats slower. If you're 46 to 55, it can be a couple of beats higher.

(*Important note*: If you get a pain in your chest, or your knees hurt, stop at once. See your GP before taking any further exercise.)

Aerobic exercise is fast-paced activity that works up a sweat and raises your heart rate till you're almost out of breath. You should get up to a level at which you can just about continue a conversation, and keep at this level for about half an hour. This aids weight loss and improves your cardiovascular fitness: your heart's ability to pump oxygenated blood around your body.

Muscle-building, including training with weights, does more than just increase your strength. You'll look your best with toned abdominal muscles holding your stomach in and the curve of muscle creating shapelier limbs. Gyms are the traditional place to work out on a range of machines that use resistance to challenge your muscles. Some classes do workouts with hand weights, or you can buy these to use at home. Any weight-bearing exercise, such as running or hiking, provides the bonus of strengthening your bones too.

Flexibility work keeps your joints mobile, reduces your risk of injury and lengthens your muscles to create smooth curves. Aerobics classes normally include a few minutes' stretching to protect the muscles, and if you join a gym you'll be taught to do the same kind of stretches before and after using the machines. Most gyms offer some kind of stretch class too.

Yoga or Pilates are two of the best methods you can use to improve flexibility, and to build and tone muscles at the same time. High-speed forms of yoga such as astanga give an all-round workout by raising your heartbeat. But these are too strenuous for most beginners: if this appeals, work your way up to it with normal yoga and aerobics classes.

It only takes a small amount of extra time to discover what you most need to work on, and how to do it most effectively. You can then create a workout regime tailored to your specific needs.

Start taking control now by finding a fitness routine that suits your way of life. You may not like the first thing you try, but don't let that put you off trying something else. If your first aerobics class leaves you wincing at the naff music, look for one that uses your kind of sound – salsa, for example, or African drumming. Join a local sports club and be part of a team. Or put on your headphones and go for a run in the park!

Keep shopping around till you settle on something you can stick with. It doesn't have to be for ever. If you started with something easy, you'll want to move on to more challenging activities as you get in shape. You'll probably find new fitness interests, as in any area of life.

Build it into your life

We've all made New Year resolutions that faded in the cold light of January, and 'Get fit' is one of the most frequently made and broken.

The only way to become and stay fit is to make exercise part of your everyday routine, as natural and inevitable as brushing your hair.

Because our body clocks affect all aspects of our daily rhythms, we're best suited to exercise at about 6 p.m. That's the time of day when our muscles are at their most supple and we have the highest levels of energy and endurance. This is handy for a visit to the gym on the way home from work. But if you feel tired, have to work late or want to meet friends, it's easy to keep missing that evening workout.

Studies have shown that, despite their body clocks, most people who work out regularly do it first thing in the morning. It's simple to set the alarm an hour earlier and get it out of the way before work or other daily commitments. Whether you do your own workout at home or drop in at the gym on the way to work, you'll feel good about it, and it will give you a blast of extra energy for the day.

Gym'll fix it

Though anyone can work out at home, it can be an uphill struggle to persevere before you get fit enough to see the benefits. Joining a gym makes it infinitely easier. Local authorities provide facilities at reasonable prices, and usually offer reduced rates if you can attend at less popular times, such as during office hours.

Paying a monthly fee provides immediate motivation for going there as often as possible. When you're starting to flag, the presence of everyone else around you adds some gentle peer pressure to continue. You may make friends there, or persuade a friend to go with you – and training with someone else is a strong motivation to keep going when you feel sluggish.

Unless you live in the most fashionable area or join a very exclusive gym, you're unlikely to find yourself surrounded by model lookalikes. Many other women there are likely to be around your own age and most will be trying to fend off the ravages of childbirth, fast food or sedentary jobs.

You can get fit using weight and cardiovascular machines. But do try some classes too – you may be surprised how much fun they are. The range and variety of activities almost guarantees you'll find something you enjoy and, importantly, being in a group keeps you going when you might have given up alone. Some classes use gym equipment such as stationary bikes, trampolines or weights machines. Others are just you and the music.

'I'd always feel better if I went to the gym'

At the front of the aerobics class in the advanced section, Sheila looks enviously young and fit to those behind struggling to keep up. Her slender curves and flat stomach don't fit anyone's idea of a post-menopausal body shape. But she cheerfully says she's 55 and 'never bothered' with HRT.

Sheila was 40 when a leaflet advertising a local gym came through her door. She hadn't taken any exercise since her four-year-old son was born.

'I walked past the door twice, thinking I can't go in there,' she says. Luckily, she pushed herself to go in. 'I started doing circuit training, weights and machines and found I really enjoyed it. I'm about the same shape now as I was then. I've got a sweet tooth, but I just seem to burn it off.'

Her toned body comes at a price: four two-hourly sessions a week of exercises, machines and classes. 'As you get older, you have to work harder to get the results, because your body gets used to it,' she says. 'You have to do a little bit extra or try something a bit different – even just changing the order you do things in. And you do have to eat less!'

But it's worth the effort, and not just to look good. Her boundless energy lets her enjoy her work as a school midday assistant, in a playground full of boisterous children, as well as playing with her grandchildren. Fit and supple, she has avoided the perimenopausal spiral of tiredness and other physical symptoms leading to reduced activity which, in turn, reduces fitness and exacerbates the symptoms.

Going through perimenopause in her forties Sheila suffered from hot flushes, heavy periods and mood swings.

'Exercise didn't stop the hot flushes, but it helped me cope,' she says. 'Also, I used to get very bad mood swings, and it definitely helped with those. I would resent it if my period was so heavy that I couldn't exercise. When I was feeling moody, I'd always feel better if I went to the gym.'

How much is enough?

How much exercise do you need to do? Unless you're already very fit, the answer is likely to be 'a bit more than you're doing now'. In other words, start with something that's a slight challenge, and work on up.

Do the step test (see box above) to see how fit you are. If you're out of condition or haven't exercised since you were at school, start by doing three half-hour fitness activities a week: a brisk walk home after getting off the bus early, a football match with the children, and some energetic housework would do it.

But don't stay at that level longer than necessary. To improve your fitness, you should soon be doing about an hour of proper exercise three or four times a week. This should include cardiovascular work, muscle-building and flexibility.

You can do all of these at home, devising a routine to suit yourself. There's now a huge range of workout videos and DVDs available. The quality is variable, though, and you can't tell from the sleek packaging how good the instructor is. If you're planning to use any of these, check their ratings in a specialist magazine such as *Health & Fitness*. Look in your local library for those the reviewers recommend if possible before buying them, to see if it's something you're likely to stick with.

If you're doing one-hour sessions, look for a class that starts with a warm-up and stretch, followed by about half an hour of aerobic exercise that ends with a brief cool-down period, then some muscle-building exercise and finally some more stretches. Most gyms offer a range of aerobics classes, many of them based on this pattern. Others will be mainly aerobic work with some stretches, or a mixture of muscle-building and stretching.

'I feel younger and fitter now than I did before the perimeno-pause'

Lucy, whose symptoms turned out to be caused by heart disease (see Chapter 2), says she went through the perimenopause in reverse gear. After a coronary bypass and a period of rehabilitation, she was advised to take regular exercise.

'I was very unfit, but I presumed I always would be now because of the heart disease,' she says. She hated the thought of gyms, so she eventually started yoga and tai chi classes. Soon she found her whole outlook was changing.

'I suppose I'd always lived in my head, never taken much care of my body,' she says. As she became stronger and more supple, her energy started increasing. She tried a beginners' aerobics class and was soon going twice a week. As her health and vitality increased over the next couple of years, she started going out more, her spirits lifted, she stopped overeating, her weight slid downwards and she became even more active.

'I'd felt old and worn out, but I realized much later that some of the symptoms were perimenopausal,' she says. 'Tripping over, for example – I just thought I was getting old! But as I got stronger and fitter, I stopped falling down, and I could run again. Tai chi helped with my balance too. My joints used to ache and feel stiff, but yoga has fixed that.

'I feel younger and fitter now than I did 15 years ago, before I had heart disease or the perimenopause.'

Safety first

- Check with your GP before starting any exercise programme, especially if you are taking medicine or have a health problem.
- Start at a level that only presents a slight challenge, and work on up as you become fitter.
- Stop at once if you feel pain, other than a slight muscle ache. Seek medical advice immediately if the pain is sharp, or in three days if a milder pain hasn't worn off, or if a pain keeps recurring.
- Don't become obsessed with formal exercise. Four or five sessions a week of classes or in the gym is plenty. Back it up by becoming more active in your everyday life too.

10
Long-term health

Many perimenopausal symptoms ease off after the menopause – an unexpected delight with those symptoms you didn't even realize were hormone-related, such as anxiety or clumsiness. Others – such as joint pains and memory loss – that you thought were signs of premature ageing, can also disappear when your hormones have found their new equilibrium. Suddenly, when you were least expecting to, you feel ten years younger.

Some of the hormonal changes that start during the perimenopause are permanent, it's true. As we've seen, you have to work harder to keep your skin and waistline in good shape, for example. But, in your thirties and forties you can still take measures to slow down the ageing process and much increase your chances of a healthy and active old age. Most of us could improve our eating habits, for example, and now is an excellent time to find healthier new ones.

Despite the hectic lives so many of us lead, we're likely to become less physically active by our late thirties – often just because there's no time for the activities that used to keep us fit. Annoyingly, running around after children or problem-solving at work don't give the kind of muscle-toning or heart-conditioning exercise we need. And when our pulses do race, it's more likely to be with stress or anxiety than as a result of healthy activity.

Adapting your lifestyle with some of the ideas in Chapters 8 and 9 will pay off both now and later. The easy changes you make now can save you from years of unnecessary discomfort during the perimenopause. And, after the menopause, they will go on repaying you for decades with vitality, youthful looks and good health.

Playing your genetic cards to win

Observe your mother and other older female relatives, on both sides of the family, for clues as to how you're likely to age. Ask questions too, bearing in mind that they've got the benefit of years more experience, and may give you advice that they wish someone had given them.

Do members of your family tend to pile on weight? Become small and hunched? Stiffen up in the joints? You're quite likely to face the same challenges, so be forewarned and take preventative action now. All of these can be kept at bay with a tailored fitness routine, backed up by healthy eating.

This is also a good time to ask about any diseases or health conditions that run in the family – you may not necessarily know, as these aren't always discussed even among relatives. Many diseases have a genetic component, including several cancers. You can reduce your risk of many of these by screening and lifestyle changes – ask your GP for more information.

Remember that your genetic inheritance is just the hand you're dealt. It's up to you whether you throw away the good cards, or win despite having been dealt an unpromising hand.

Reducing your risks

After the menopause, you're at increased risk of heart disease, osteoporosis and certain cancers. The risks increase sharply if you do nothing to avoid them, but much less so if you started preventative action in good time.

Heart disease

Although young women are not immune to coronary heart disease, it is quite unusual in non-smokers who are still menstruating. The menopause puts an end to your hormones' protective influence on your blood vessels, and your risk of hardened arteries, heart attacks and strokes quickly increases to roughly the same as a man's risk.

Despite our fears about breast cancer, heart disease actually kills more women. Luckily, it is one of the easiest diseases to have some control over.

The most effective action you can take is to stop smoking. The earlier you do this, the less your arteries will be damaged and the faster and more completely they will heal.

Almost as important is stress. It's long been known to exacerbate existing heart disease, and increase the risk of a heart attack in people already at risk. But researchers are now starting to believe that healthy people put themselves at risk of developing heart disease if they're under prolonged stress.

In fact, emotional factors are increasingly being recognized as playing a vital role, for good and bad, in physical health. Long-standing depression, for example, can increase your risk of serious diseases such as heart disease and possibly cancer. (See Chapter 3 for ways of coping with stress and depression.)

Healthy eating plays a vital role in maintaining heart health, so try to replace snacks and sweets with nuts and fruit, and put more vegetables on your plate at every meal. A low-fat diet is believed to reduce the build-up of cholesterol in the coronary arteries, but not all fats are equal. Your heart will benefit if you eat oily fish twice a week and cook with vegetable oils, which also make tasty salad dressings when mixed with vinegar or lemon juice. Saturated fats are what you should avoid, and worst of all for your heart are trans-fats (see box below).

Trans-fats

Created in the hydrogenation process that makes oils solid at room temperature, these prolong the shelf-life of sweets, cakes, biscuits and numerous other processed foods. Commercial deep-fried foods also contain transfats – the more often the oil is reused, the higher the trans-fat content. Unlike the vegetable oils they're usually made from, they're a form of saturated fat, implicated in heart disease by raising the amount of LDL, or bad cholesterol, in our blood. Many researchers believe they are more harmful than other saturated fats: a paper published in the *Lancet* in 2001 claimed that reducing our intake of trans-fats by 2.4 per cent could cut the death toll from heart disease by a quarter.

You can avoid trans-fats by not buying fried foods and by stir-frying instead of deep-frying at home. Cut down on bought pastries, cakes, biscuits and any product with 'shortening' or 'hydrogenated' on the label – for example, in 'partially hydrogenated vegetable oil'. And eat organic products: they're not allowed to contain hydrogenated fats.

You may have an increased risk of heart disease if:

- Coronary heart disease or high cholesterol runs in your family.
- You have high blood pressure.
- You have diabetes.
- You had an early menopause, whether this was natural or caused by hysterectomy or chemotherapy.
- You smoke.

- You have ever been severely underweight – for example, through anorexia.
- You eat a lot of processed foods.
- You are often very stressed or unhappy.

Osteoporosis

Poor bone density can lead to osteoporosis, the brittle-bone condition that causes fractures and spinal deformities. Osteoporosis usually affects older people, especially women, but its effects can start to be felt much earlier if your bones are vulnerable. Eating disorders are the best-known cause in young women, but a sedentary life increases your risk.

Are you at risk for osteoporosis?

You may have an increased risk of osteoporosis if:

- Your mother, sister, aunt or grandmother has it.
- You're Asian – black women have the lowest risk, and white women are in between.
- You're underweight.
- You've often crash-dieted.
- You're small-boned.
- You ever stopped having periods except during pregnancy or the perimenopause.
- You've never been pregnant.
- You had an early menopause.
- You lead a sedentary life.
- You smoke or drink alcohol.
- You use certain medicines every day, such as steroids (say for asthma) and thyroid drugs. Diuretics and indigestion remedies containing aluminium also steal the calcium you need to keep your bones strong.

Until your late thirties you can build up your bone density through weight-bearing exercise. Once you pass 40, your bones no longer build strength; in fact, they're already starting to lose their density. The work you do after that age is to try to slow down the bone-thinning process. So it's vital to build them up as much as possible before the end of your thirties.

To build strong bones you need calcium (see Chapter 8 for sources) and Vitamin D. As with all nutrients, it's better to get these in their natural form rather than as food supplements, which can easily upset the fine balance of nutrients in your body.

Vitamin D is made from sunshine: your body produces this nutrient through the effects of sun on your skin. And as walking is one of the best defences against osteoporosis, don't hide from the sun all the time. In the early morning and late afternoon, and during the winter, its rays aren't strong enough to harm you and getting some sun on your skin will do you nothing but good.

Cancers

Cancer isn't just one disease: the many different kinds of cancer have many different causes. Those of the reproductive system, and especially womb and breast cancer, are encouraged to grow by oestrogen, which is why doctors are cautious about offering HRT if you or a close relative has had one of these cancers.

For this reason, it's important to check your breasts for lumps, and be aware of any other bodily changes – for example, excessive bleeding or back pain – that won't go away. Take advantage of any screening programmes: don't miss your regular mammograms and smear tests. In case you're not sent an appointment by your GP or local health authority, keep a note of when you last had either of these tests so you can remind them.

There is also increasing evidence that we are affected by xenoestrogens, hormone-disrupting chemicals spread through our environment by pollution. Some of these can't be avoided, as they're in the very air we breathe. But we can reduce our exposure to many of them (see Chapter 1).

These are not the only cancers we are more likely to face as we get older. The most dangerous form of skin cancer, malignant melanoma, is rapidly becoming more common. That's partly due to environmental damage: widespread use of aerosols has torn a hole in the ozone layer that used to protect people from the harmful rays of the sun. But we've also had several decades of cheap holidays in sunny climates – irresistible but dangerous to those of European ancestry whose skin has adapted to cloudy northern skies.

Everyone who has ever had sunburn, especially before the age of 20, is now warned to look out for the signs of skin cancer. But there's increasing evidence that it could strike people who haven't had sunburn, and of course few of us would remember if we were sunburnt in early childhood.

Skin cancers are easy to remove in the early stages, so it makes sense for everyone to check now and then. Look out for moles that grow larger, change in shape (especially to develop irregular outlines), or become darker. Because they often grow on parts of the body that are covered up till we hit the beaches, they're frequently found on legs and backs – areas that aren't easy to see – so share a regular mole check with your partner or a close friend.

Bowel cancer often develops after years of constipation, so a high-fibre diet can reduce your risk. But there's rarely a need to eat special foods for their high fibre content: a healthy diet based on fruit and vegetables should have the same effect more naturally.

In fact, it's impossible to list the number of health conditions, especially cancers, that are less likely to develop in someone who eats a healthy diet. Practically every month, new research is published showing the amazing health-promoting benefits of some fruit or vegetable. It's pretty much all true – these nutritional powerhouses are the healthiest ingredients anyone can eat, packed with nutrients that have never been copied into a drug or distilled into a vitamin pill. And of all their disease-fighting properties, none are more highly valued than their ability to reduce the risk of many cancers.

You may have an increased risk of cancer if:

● You don't eat enough fruit and vegetables.
● You have a poor diet generally.
● You had certain infections when you were young, including sexually transmitted diseases.
● It runs in your family.
● You smoke.
● You work with chemicals or other hazardous substances.
● You work in a poorly ventilated office: some office equipment gives off fumes that can build up.

You may have an increased risk of breast cancer if:

● Your mother, sister, aunt or grandmother had it.
● You have benign breast disease (such as fibrocystic breast changes – non-cancerous lumps).
● You had a first pregnancy after the age of 30.
● You drink more than three units of alcohol a day.
● You are overweight.

The shape of things to come?

If you look at women in their late forties and beyond, you notice that the changes aren't just about putting on weight: a woman's entire silhouette subtly alters. It's a process that can start as early as your thirties if you haven't been taking care of yourself. Luckily, at this stage it is still largely reversible.

Oestrogen is the hormone that gives women of child-bearing age their distinctive curvy shape. As children we had straighter outlines, as do men and old people in their different ways. At puberty all that changes. Allowing for the vast range of normal body shapes and sizes, most women of child-bearing age have relatively small waists, large hips and noticeable breasts. We tend to put extra weight on our hips and thighs, accentuating that feminine shape.

As oestrogen levels drop, your curves start to flatten out. Weight creeps on to your stomach and abdomen, where you'd never seen it before. Changes in your metabolism mean that you need a little less food than before. Without eating a mouthful more or taking any less exercise, you will slowly gain weight if you don't take action to avoid it.

Your breasts sink lower on your chest and the tissue becomes softer and less dense. Even if you don't put on weight, your waist becomes less defined. In addition, your muscles lose tone, so your upper arms become flabby and your buttocks droop. Even your bone structure is affected: what looks at first like round shoulders may be the beginning of a 'dowager's hump'. That's an early sign of poor bone density, leading to osteoporosis. In addition, low oestrogen levels mean your skin is drier and membranes are less lubricated than before.

It wouldn't be worth saying all this just to depress you. The good news is that it doesn't have to happen. Without making foolish claims about stopping the ageing process, you can delay some of these changes and reduce or even prevent others. It's not even difficult or time-consuming.

Take a look at elderly yoga teachers, sportswomen and others who've stayed fit as either a side effect or a condition of their career. Consider those stupendous fashion models and actresses in their sixties, and older, who walk and move like much younger women. They may have been born pretty – or had cosmetic surgery – but that's not why they still look good now. It's their bodies, rather than their faces, that have held back time. There's nothing miraculous about it. They've just built fitness into their everyday lives.

Keeping your looks is a powerful motivation. And that's fortunate, because those seemingly superficial alterations may be the outward sign of deteriorating health.

Becoming overweight puts you at risk of diabetes. The thickening of your waist, giving you a more masculine 'beer-belly' outline, increases your risk of heart disease. Healthy eating and aerobic exercise keep your overall weight under control, while muscle-toning exercises reduce the appearance of a spare tyre. (See Chapters 8 and 9 for details.)

Aerobic exercise has beneficial effects on your skin too, by improving its oxygen supply. And the biggest motivation for eating healthily is your skin's visible response to better nutrition.

As mentioned above, an incipient 'dowager's hump' shows that you're at risk of osteoporosis. This is easier to prevent than to cure, with a diet high in calcium and other nutrients that help your body use the calcium to build bone. Weight-bearing exercise is equally important (see Chapter 9).

Those round shoulders are also compressing your chest, reducing your lung capacity and therefore your oxygen supply. The easiest way to tackle this is to improve your posture (see Chapter 9). Breathing exercises, usually practised for their calming effects, can also improve your respiratory function (see Chapter 7).

Loss of muscle tone puts you at risk of falls and injuries. Weight-bearing exercise and workouts to build specific muscles will counteract this. As a bonus, building muscle improves your skin tone as well as your shape. Tai chi, yoga and qi gong can all improve your sense of balance, and their meditative movements could soothe tension lines out of your face. Taking action to stay in shape will keep you looking as well as feeling young, and ward off some of the major health risks of old age.

'Maybe I've been lucky, but the way I live helps'
If you saw Ilse running down the street ahead of you, you'd never guess her age. Close up, her face admits that's she's over 70 and the fair hair piled on her head is actually white. But her spine is unbent and her movements are as graceful as a dancer's.

'I've never worried much about my health,' she says. 'Luckily I haven't needed to. I gave up smoking when I was still young – actually, it was when I took up yoga, and that's a few decades ago now! And I don't eat rubbish. I never have, I just don't like it. I've always enjoyed cooking, proper meals with fresh meat and vegetables, even when I was busy, so I suppose I've had a pretty healthy diet. I eat a lot less meat now than I used to, but I couldn't quite go vegetarian.'

A retired office administrator, Ilse is active in community groups and spends much of her free time gardening or visiting museums and art galleries with friends. In fact, she says she is busier in many ways than when she was employed.

One thing she makes time for every day is her yoga practice. She starts each morning with a series of moves that work all parts of her body, tailored to her age. 'When I was going through the menopause I started doing more of the standing poses and ones that strengthen your arms, because I wanted to keep my bones strong – I was a bit worried about getting osteoporosis. I also do a lot of walking. I've never owned a car.'

Despite a healthy lifestyle, she admits she was a sun-worshipper in her youth – 'we all were in those days' – and only changed her ways after having an early-stage skin cancer cut out. She now has regular check-ups and covers up in the sun.

'Maybe I've been lucky – some of my friends have died, of heart disease and cancer, and they didn't live particularly unhealthy lives. But I think the way I live helps, and I've had a chance to do things I like.'

Good times ahead

If you're already noticing some perimenopausal symptoms, the view ahead may look bleak. More heavy periods or hot flushes till the menopause is over, then everything else getting worse as old age takes over.

The good news is, that's not the case – it gets better! The trouble with such well-known signs of the perimenopause is that people don't realize they're not the only symptoms that are temporary.

Other disturbances, such as poor memory, joint pains, confusion and clumsiness, are often far more upsetting – especially when they're gloomily accepted as the first signs of old age. Yet the hormones governing your menstrual cycles, especially oestrogen, also have an effect on your brain and central nervous system. And when they settle into a new balance after menopause, you may be amazed at how many of your old capacities come back.

Many women actually feel better after the menopause than they did a decade earlier, and not just compared to the perimenopausal years. Those who always had heavy or painful periods gain a new

111

lease of life once their menstrual cycles stop. Fibroids and endometriosis are no longer a problem.

Less predictably, several health conditions ease after the menopause even though they weren't obviously linked with reproductive hormones. Many migraine sufferers enjoy freedom from their crippling headaches after the menopause. Allergies often clear up too. Women suffer less depression after the menopause than before, and even serious mental illness such as schizophrenia can be relieved.

If you've started building optimal health before the menopause, you may well find that you feel fitter and happier afterwards than ever before!

Useful addresses

Arthritis Research Campaign
Copeman House
St Mary's Court
St Mary's Gate
Chesterfield
Derbyshire S41 7TD
Tel.: 0870 850 5000
Website: www.arc.org.uk
Email: info@arc.org.uk

Includes osteoporosis.

Baby Cafes
www.thebabycafe.co.uk

Informative site for breastfeeding mothers.

Breastfeeding Network
PO Box 11126
Paisley PA2 8YB
Scotland
National helpline 0870 900 8787
Website: www.breastfeedingnetwork.org.uk
Email: bfn@btinternet.com

British Association for Behavioural and Cognitive Psychotherapies
The Globe Centre
PO Box 9
Accrington BB5 0XB
Tel.: 01254 875277
Website: www.babcp.com
Email: babcp@babcp.com

British Complementary Medicine Association
PO Box 5122
Bournemouth BH8 0WG
Tel.: 0845 345 5977
Website: www.bcma.co.uk
Email: info@bcma.co.uk

British Heart Foundation
14 Fitzhardinge Street
London W1H 6DH
Tel.: 08450 70 80 70 (Heart Information Line)
Website: www.bhf.org.uk
Email: internet@bhf.org.uk

British Wheel of Yoga
25 Jermyn Street
Sleaford
Lincolnshire NG34 7RU
Tel.: 01529 306851
Website: www.bwy.org.uk
Email: office@bwy.org.uk

Family Planning Association
Information Department
2–12 Pentonville Road
London N1 9FP
Tel.: 0845 310 1334 (Monday to Friday, 9 a.m. to 6 p.m.)
Website: www.fpa.org.uk

Fertility UK
Bury Knowle Health Centre
207 London Road
Headington
Oxford OX3 9JA
Website: www.fertilityuk.org
Email:admin@fertilityuk.org

Natural family planning and fertility advice.

The Human Givens Institute
Chalvington
East Sussex BN27 3TD
Tel.: 01323 811662
Website: www.humangivens.com/hgi
Email: hgi@humangivens.com

Institute for Complementary Medicine (ICM)
PO Box 194
London SE16 7QZ
Tel.: 020 7237 5165
Website: www.i-c-m.org.uk
Email: info@i-c-m.org.uk

Jane's Breastfeeding Resources
Website: www.breastfeeding.co.uk

A site dealing with news, resources, articles and questions on breastfeeding.

National Childbirth Trust
Alexandra House
Oldham Terrace
London W3 6NH
Tel.: 0870 444 8707 (Enquiries Line)
      08709 90 8040 (Membership Line)
Website: www.nctpregnancyandbabycare.com
Email: enquiries@national-childbirth-trust.co.uk

National Health Service
24-hour helplines 0845 46 47 (England and Wales), 08454 24 24 24 (Scotland)
Website: www.nhs.uk
NHS information website: www.besttreatments.co.uk

National Register of Personal Trainers
PO Box 314
Chalfont St Peter
Buckinghamshire SL9 9ZL
Tel.: 0870 200 6010
Website: www.nrpt.co.uk

Register of Exercise Professionals
Website: www.exerciseregister.org/check-out-your-instructor.htm

Soil Association
Bristol House
40–56 Victoria Street
Bristol BS1 6BY
Tel.: 0117 314 5000
Website: www.soilassociation.org
Email: info@soilassociation.org

Women's Health
52 Featherstone Street
London EC1Y 8RT
Tel.: 0845 125 5254 (Monday to Friday: 9.30 a.m.–1.30 p.m.
Website: www.womenshealthlondon.org.uk

Women's Nutritional Advisory Service
PO Box 268
Lewes
East Sussex BN7 1QN
Tel.: 09062 556615
Website: www.naturalhealthas.com
Email: enquiries@naturalhealthas.com

The Yoga Biomedical Trust
9–92 Pentonville Road
London N1 9HS
Tel.: 020 7689 3040
Website: www.yogatherapy.org
Email: enquiries.yogatherapy@virgin.net

YMCA Sports Centres

England
Website:www.ymca.org.uk

Wales
Website: www.ymca-wales.org
Email: contact@ymca-wales.org

Scotland
Website: www.ymcascotland.org
Email: info@ymcascotland.org

Ireland
Website: www.ymca-ireland.org
Email: admin@ymca-ireland.org

Further reading

Health & Fitness magazine, *solutions@hfonline.co.uk*
www.hfonline.co.uk

The Change Before the Change, by Dr Laura E. Corio and Linda G. Kahn, Piatkus 2002. A big book, written from the medical angle but with plenty of other information too. Written before the negative results of the latest HRT studies were known.

Help Your Child Get Fit not Fat, by Jan Hurst & Sue Hubberstey, Sheldon Press, 2005.

Ayurveda for Beauty and Health, by Janet Wright, Southwater, 2005.

Beat Menopause Naturally, by Maryon Stewart, Natural Health Advisory Service, 2003. The nutritional angle, recommending supplements. This is also an e-book: see http://www.naturalcures 4menopause.com/nc4m/UK/bmn-ebook1.htm

Hot Flashes, Warm Bottles: First-Time Mothers over Forty, by Nancy London, Celestial Arts, 2001.

What Your Doctor May Not Tell You About Premenopause, by John R. Lee, Jesse Hanley and Virginia Hopkins, Warner, 1999. The case for supplementing with progesterone. Written before the negative results of the latest HRT studies were known.

Index

term health 103–4; signs and
symptoms 4–7, 9–11;
symptoms from other causes
15–16; temporary symptoms
111–12
periods: bleeding and cancer 12;
changes in 4; exercise and
fitness 93; foods for 88–90;
hormonal cycle 8–9; HRT
and 57–8; other problems
16–17; symptoms of
perimenopause 6
phytoestrogens 62–3, 86
Pilates 98
the Pill: contraception 32–3;
health risks 33; as HRT 59
pregnancy 1; fertility 10–11;
later years 31–2; miscarriage
40; older mothers and 39–40
premenstrual syndrome (PMS) 4,
17, 22; herbal remedies 68
progesterone 57–8; changes at
perimenopause 7–9; natural
65–6
progestogens 51
psychotherapy 25–6, 28

red clover 64
rheumatoid arthritis 10

St John's Wort 68
selective serotonin-reuptake
inhibitors (SSRIs) 58–9
sex drive: decrease in 6, 22,
26–7; fertility and 36–7; new
mothers 46
sexually-transmitted diseases:

fertility and 35; symptoms 18
skin: ageing of 18–19; cancer
107–8; dryness 5
sleep apnoea 21
stress 23
strokes 54
suicide risk 24–5

testosterone 58
thrush 6, 18, 69, 90
thyroid disorder 17; symptoms
of 19
Tibolone 58
tiredness 1, 5; foods for 87;
from heavy bleeding 46; other
causes 21; sex life and 26
Trifolium pratense 64–5

urinary system: diet and
nutrition 90; incontinence 6,
72–4; infections 6, 18, 68–9
uterine cancer 11; oestrogens
and 50–2

vaginal dryness 17–18, 57
Vitex agnus castus 65

weight: ageing shapes 109–10;
BMI 83, 85; change of shape
19; fertility and 35; gaining
6, 10; nutrition and 82–5;
slowed metabolism 18–19
Wilson, Dr Robert A. 50

yams, wild or Mexican 65
yoga 98